Elizabeth T. Hall

Caring for a Loved One with Alzheimer's Disease
A Christian Perspective

"**W**e cannot understand Alzheimer's disease unless we really live it. This book schools us in what to watch for, how to try to understand what is happening, and ways to try to cope through tougher and tougher situations. In these essays we find the reality of what the disease means for the loved ones dealing with it daily. This book itself is Velma's story, the story of Alzheimer's and what it has done to Velma. But it is also the story of a lone woman dedicated to her family and doing whatever is necessary to care for them. The author's heartfelt essays about her deepest thoughts and emotions tell the story of what it is to live with Alzheimer's as the person who understands what is happening (as the patient clearly does not). In these essays, we get the true feeling of the anger, fear, empathy, and ultimate faith in God involved in caring for a loved one with Alzheimer's. I know this book will speak to others who have the same task and will remind them that God is able when we cast our cares on Him and ask Him to bear our very heavy burdens."

Jean Archambault-White
Durham, North Carolina

The Haworth Pastoral Press
An Imprint of The Haworth Press, Inc.

Caring for a Loved One with Alzheimer's Disease

A Christian Perspective

THE HAWORTH PASTORAL PRESS
Religion and Mental Health
Harold G. Koenig, MD
Senior Editor

New, Recent, and Forthcoming Titles:

Caring for a Loved One with Alzheimer's Disease
A Christian Perspective

Elizabeth T. Hall

The Haworth Pastoral Press
An Imprint of The Haworth Press, Inc.
New York • London • Oxford

Published by

The Haworth Pastoral Press, an imprint of The Haworth Press, Inc., 10 Alice Street, Binghamton, NY 13904-1580

Cover design by Marylouise E. Doyle.

Library of Congress Cataloging-in-Publication Data

Hall, Elizabeth T. (Elizabeth Thomason), 1941-
    Caring for a loved one with Alzheimer's disease : a Christian perspective / Elizabeth T. Hall.
      p. cm.
    Includes bibliographical references and index.
    ISBN 0-7890-0872-6 (alk. paper).—ISBN 0-7890-0873-4 (pbk. : alk. paper)
     1. Caregivers—Religious life. 2. Alzheimer's disease—Religious aspects—Christianity. 3. Hall, Elizabeth T. (Elizabeth Thomason), 1941- . I. Title.
BV4910.9.H35 2000
259′.4196831—dc21
                                                      99-37685
                                                     CIP

For Jordan

ABOUT THE AUTHOR

Elizabeth T. Hall, BS, is a native of West Tennessee. She has been caring for her mother, Velma Thomason, since the onset of aging disabilities, loss of vision, and severe arthritis. She has published an article titled "I Don't Want to Be a Caregiver," published in *The Caregiver,* Duke University's Family Support Group newsletter. She has been involved in family support groups, spoken on the topic of caregiving, and continues to be an advocate for both the patient and the family suffering the depredations of this dreaded disease.

CONTENTS

My Statement of Faith

This I believe, as did the early Church fathers. I believe that God has not changed since He walked in the garden and communed with Adam and Eve and that only our own sin and failure to learn to know Him in His glory stands in the way of our communion with Him. He is the strength of my life in the dark hours, my glory, and the lifter of my head.

If this volume ended with this statement it would explain wholly how I have been able to deal with my mother's illness and give the glory to the One who made it possible.

As we have walked through this disease process together I have been sustained by "Yea, though I walk through the valley of the shadow of death, I will fear no evil: for Thou art with me; thy rod and thy staff they comfort me" (Psalms 23:4, KJV).

The senile dementias are truly the "valley of the shadow" and the valley is long. I know as we walk that we are not alone and that He truly walks beside us and when the load becomes too heavy He carries us. In the midst of despair He comforts us and will be there at the end of our walk to receive us unto Himself.

Preface

This volume is not intended to be a scholarly tome giving all the answers needed for family members dealing with loved ones suffering from a dementing illness. It is one daughter's story of her mother's long journey from normalcy through the various stages of dementia. It is written from pain, despair, acceptance, and victory. It is written from an ever more intimate knowledge of my Lord, Jesus Christ, without whom each step would have been more than I could bear. It is written in the hope that, through my experiences, other family members dealing with dementia may avoid some of the pitfalls I experienced and find peace sooner than I did.

I do not pretend to have all the answers. Indeed, as time goes by I realize that I do not even know all the questions. In fact this volume raises many more questions than it answers. However, through it all, I have learned more truly than ever before that the God of the mountain also walks the valley with us. Throughout the ordeal, whatever the trial, I have learned to lean ever more heavily on God's grace. I have found that, indeed, His grace is sufficient.

Nevertheless, the arduous journey has been both mind-numbing and nerve-racking as we stumble through trial and error in treatment, living arrangements, decision making, and getting reacquainted after each personality change.

Even after learning to lean on Him, there have been days when frustration and despair were my constant companions. Many times I have cried out to Him in hurt and anger, reminding that He promised that His yoke would be easy and His burden light. Always He answers, in the kind, loving way that only He can:

"Then let me carry it awhile." I have learned to listen for God's voice in the midst of trials I could not have borne in earlier years. I have learned that prayer is a two-way communication and that I must spend more time listening than talking.

I have no idea how a family could begin to deal with the pain, despair, and confusion inherent in a dementing illness without the grace, wisdom, and strength of God to draw upon. Viewing this disease from a Christian perspective is the only possible way I could have started my "walk through the valley" several years ago and to be stronger for it after each trial.

Thank God also that along with strength and grace He blesses me with a sense of humor, which lightens the daily burdens, and that, after the early years of fear, He has restored my mother's sense of humor.

As my mother and I continue our journey through the valley of the shadow of death I realize more fully that God is preparing me for the ministry of my mature years, and that He knew I needed the training. I realize that He has led me a long way (*all* the way so far) in my journey through life, until I have finally reached the point where I realize that I have no one but Him to turn to in life's darkest hours.

Acknowledgments

My most heartfelt thanks go to Anthony Galanos, MD, my mother's physician, who has walked through this valley with us; Diane Wildman, social worker at Duke's Geriatric Evaluation and Treatment Center, upon whom I have leaned heavily for support; Harold Koenig, MD, my friend and inspiration; Conrad Fulkerson, MD, my psychiatrist; and David Bowman, my pastor, who all have served as inspirations to keep the faith and who have all encouraged me in my efforts both to care for my mother and to write about this experience. Thanks also to Priscilla Finch, Jean White, Susan Bowman, and Lynn Robbins, my best friends and sisters in the Lord who have borne me up during the tough times with prayers, encouragement, and practical help; to Betty Stephenson, my co-worker and friend who listened and let me cry on her shoulder; and to Edna Ballard and Cornelia Poer of Duke University's family support group where I can go when I feel most alone.

Special thanks go to my sons Richard, Greg, and Jim, their wives Karen, Tina, and Colleen, and my grandson, Matthew, simply for being there and letting a little sunshine in on the darkest days, for providing respite when my mind and my body could stand no more, and laughter when life seems darkest.

Most of all, thanks to my mother, Velma Thomason, with whom I have walked hand in hand through this long dark night of the soul and who still loves me through all my mistakes—even on days when she doesn't remember who I am.

The Apostles' Creed

I believe in God the Father Almighty, Maker of Heaven
and Earth
And in Jesus Christ, His Only Son, our Lord
Who was conceived of the Holy Spirit,
Born of the Virgin Mary,
Suffered under Pontius Pilate,
Was crucified dead and buried.
The third day He arose from the dead,
He ascended into Heaven and sitteth at the right hand of God,
The Father Almighty,
From thence He shall come to judge the quick and the dead.
I believe in the Holy Spirit,
The holy Catholic church,
The communion of saints,
The forgiveness of sins,
The resurrection of the body and life everlasting.
Amen

The Methodist Hymnal

Introduction

The Reason for It All

Alzheimer's disease comes silently, like little cat's feet, except that cat's feet are soft, loving, and remembering—not harsh, disrupting, and destroying. It is such a deceiving, disorienting, "first you see it, now you don't" kind of disease that defining when and where it strikes is almost impossible. It hides its depredations behind behaviors associated with many other diseases and behind behaviors already a part of the patient's personality so that it is in full flower before recognized as the devourer it truly is. It is our task as caregivers to make sure that we define the limits between the disease and the person for whom we care. We must never despise the person, we must always despise and fight the disease.

Our family's loss began—when? When did we first begin to notice that all was not well with Mother? She had been the heart of the family since my divorce. At a time when I was forced by circumstances to become both mother and father to my sons, spending great amounts of time simply making a living, she moved in and cared for the children. Because of emotional problems in her earlier life, she had burdened me with the chores of the protection, decision making, and major battles in my early childhood. But now she had taken charge of the practical side of our home. She laundered my children's clothing, she prepared their meals, she drove them to baseball, basketball, soccer, and football practice (as long as she was able) and managed the light housework. House and car repairs, business decisions, discipline of the children were left to me. She was always there when we came home to listen to our troubles or our triumphs. She sympathized with us in frustrations in our daily lives.

She had always preferred that we remain "loners" as far as other social events were concerned. For her the family was all important and there was no room for outsiders in our lives.

When then did we begin to notice that her behavior was not just "more so" but "different?" Was it when she became fixated on home shopping networks on TV to the exclusion of all other interests? Was it when she began to forget to launder that special shirt for a date that night? Was it when she began to burn food consistently? Was it when she ranted and raved if I made plans to attend a club meeting or to visit a friend, was it when she attempted to push a car uphill out of our driveway when she didn't want visitors?

I think that my first inkling (quickly squashed into the closet in my brain labeled "Denial") was when she stopped speaking to a doctor in our church whom she had formerly loved dearly. Her reason was that he had a bumper sticker on his vehicle speaking of Alzheimer's research. She told me that he was obviously watching her because he thought she had Alzheimer's disease. This was the farthest thing from his mind, but I couldn't convince her that he simply cherished and loved the company of older adults. Did she perhaps know even then that something was going wrong? Something none of her family and friends were ready to acknowledge?

She began to have hallucinations about famous people visiting her in our home or being invited to the White House for dinner with the President.

We, the family, knowing at last that something was dreadfully wrong, were still not ready to face *that* phrase. We discussed the possibility of a light stroke from which she would recover, we discussed circulatory problems, which could be helped by surgery.

This, then, was the point when we realized that she must be evaluated and diagnosed. We accepted in advance such things as brain tumor, cancer, or stroke, but never *that* phrase—never *Alzheimer's disease.*

And that's when the story truly began. We walked through the valley of the shadow of death with increasing dependence on a loving God who always met us at the point of our need. He has been present through the mistakes, the despair, and the helplessness has shown Himself strong in our behalf through it all. He has brought us through the stages from despair to acceptance and finally to victory over the horror of it all.

Thanks be to God for His love and care.

Chapter 1

Faith in Spite of Fear

Now faith is the substance of things hoped for, the evidence of things not seen.

Hebrews 11:1 (KJV)

As your parent, spouse, or other family member begins to exhibit personality changes, they may be so small as to be ignored or, as in my case, simply a magnification of prior habits. They do not seem important enough to be more than normal irritants of the day, nothing that really requires focused attention or changes in lifestyle. You will become irritated when he or she tells you the same story over and over. You will become more irritated when you answer the same question ten times in as many minutes. You will still probably not be ready to acknowledge that a progressive, irreversible disease process is at work and will believe that he or she could change if only he or she would pay attention.

When did my mother first exhibit signs of approaching dementia? I'm not sure. I noticed a withdrawal from friendships, but did not realize it was part of a disease process. She had always been a "loner" so her withdrawal seemed unimportant. I remembered that most of the visitors to our home in my childhood were friends of my father's rather than hers. She began to resent the friendships I had. I was an extrovert, she an introvert.

I attributed her attitude to jealousy. She had never cared for the idea of my having close friends. I ceased to invite my friends to my home and visited them in theirs. I took her out to dinner and shopping when my teenage son was having his "Super Bowl Sundays" in our home. She resented having teenage boys sitting on "her" couch and eating at "her" table. I told myself that she was beginning to resent her increasing dependency on me. She could no longer drive, she began to burn food when she cooked, she began to put toothpaste in the refrigerator and whipped cream in the medicine cabinet. She began to tell us of things she had seen on television that weren't possible. She forgot to give us messages. She forgot birthdays, especially mine. She began to call me at work each day to tell me that I had received mail and should come home at once to open it. She told us of dinners at the White House with the Carters and visits in her home from Patty Davis (President Reagan's daughter). Each new strangeness was looked upon with "after all, she's getting old." We were able to shrug off this odd behavior by thinking that she had difficulty seeing, hearing, and that memory lapses were common for the elderly. We refused to realize that memory loss to this degree is not normal.

The first real indication of a personality change was her behavior at Christmas. She had always been very generous with her gifts for the family, but now became miserly. Christmas shopping became a nightmare as she complained about the price of everything. The last Christmas I attempted to take her shopping she had bought something for everyone even though she complained. Finally she asked what I wanted. I was so exhausted with the whole procedure that I looked around where I stood, saw a pretty hot dish mat and said "How about this?" She looked at the price, $1.99, and said that she hadn't planned to spend that much for me. I felt that she thought I was too worthless to be given a gift and was hurt beyond measure. I thought, in my heart of hearts, that my years of devotion and care for her and the rest of the family were totally unappreciated. I did not receive a gift from her that year, nor have I since. I now understand that her present personality is one that doesn't recognize me as her daughter, but as her caregiver. However, each Christmas morning I feel a momentary stab of hurt before remembering that she gave me the gift of life and cared for me when I was as helpless as she is now. I realize now that her perceptions have so changed that she is incapable of being aware of the feelings of anyone around her. Her mental state resembles an infant who can only perceive her needs and wants regardless of the surroundings.

It was during this time that my own clinical depression became so severe that I began therapy. I feel sure that in the midst of my own misery I failed to notice some of hers. I believe that this was certainly the reason I misunderstood her miserliness. Looking back, I'm sure that she was suffering from depression also as she realized more and more that her cognitive functions were failing. Her depression manifested itself as anger, so I responded in the same manner.

She became ultrapossessive and very vocal about my leaving her to go anywhere other than work. She nagged me each week about my therapy and called it self-indulgent and "silly." Mother's greatest term of condemnation was always "silly." Being "silly" and being sinful were equal in her eyes. At this stage in her disease process everything not concerning her directly was "silly."

I felt that with the sense of excessive privacy she had always exhibited she probably resented my telling an "outsider" family secrets. I didn't realize that she was much past being aware of that aspect of my treatment. She was exhibiting fear and jealousy of an "other" being a part of my life. She wanted me to talk only to her. She interrupted all my conversations with my son if she was able.

She became very jealous of my friends and refused to stay in the room if they visited and insisted that I cut off phone conversations. Again, this was not new behavior, merely magnified. I was so accustomed to her attitude of "me and my wife, my son

John and his wife, us four and no more" that I hardly realized that it was a part of the disease process. I knew that I had been, in her mind, the one standing between her and hurtful or frightening experiences since my childhood. In some measure she had felt that I, even as a child, was able to solve her problems and protect her from emotions she couldn't deal with. Not realizing, again, the disease process we were faced with, and being so depressed myself, I merely attempted to discuss it with her in a calm and rational manner. She refused to discuss it other than to tell me that I was a "bad daughter" or a "bad mother." I eventually realized that I was finally, truly, the only one standing between her and the many fears she faced. This was extremely difficult for me; I had as many fears as she did and mine were real; no monsters under the bed or bad guys tapping on the windows. I now realized the truth of the verse at the beginning of this chapter. Indeed my faith was not based on anything I could see but was the substance of my hope that things would get better—either she would improve or I would learn to deal with her illness.

And I have learned, little by little, that my faith was not unfounded, but God did teach me to deal with each circumstance as it arose. Of course I made many mistakes in the early years, which I will recount and hope that you, the reader, will follow the suggestions listed rather than "muddling through" as I did.

When you, as the family member most likely to become primary caregiver, begin to suspect or to wonder if a disease process is at work, schedule a complete physical and mental evaluation with a geriatric specialist. This complete workup may constitute several visits and involve everything from chemical analysis of the blood and urine to cognitive function studies, along with a complete family history. You, as the family member, will be interviewed also and comparisons made between your interview and your relative's. Do not be surprised if your view of the family dynamic and your loved one's are not the same. I recall being aghast at my mother telling me of an answer she had given in her family history that was an outright lie. When I asked her why she had done this, her answer was that it was none of anyone's business what her childhood was like. I could not absorb the idea that she did not realize the importance of this interview to her health and treatment.

Then, after all the tests, the time will finally come when you will be scheduled to see her physician(s) and receive the diagnosis. Instead of going into this interview blindly with visions of a "magic pill" or surgical procedure that might help, the following tips will help you to survive the initial shock. These are recommendations—things I wish I had done.

1. If you have any suspicions that Alzheimer's disease may be the diagnosis, *study, study, study.* Alzheimer's is a progressive, irreversible, neurological disorder. Go to your local libraries and read everything available to you so that you can ask intelligent questions.   ˙

2. Bring in outside emotional help for yourself prior to going for the diagnosis. Ask your pastor, church care group, best friends, and so on to join in prayer with and for you, especially on the day scheduled for your physician's visit.

3. Do not go alone with your loved one to the physician's office (this learned the hard way). Take along a supportive friend or family member in the event that you are too distraught to drive home or to deal with your loved one's questions and fears.

4. Alert the family that the diagnosis is coming. Be sure to include everyone concerned. If any dementing disease is the diagnosis, do not be surprised at the variety of reactions from family members. Some may be able to handle it quite well, while others may go into a form of denial.

My family was one in which display of any emotion had been discouraged for several generations. It was surprising to me just how many were in tears when the diagnosis was made. It mattered not at all whether it was Alzheimer's disease or multi-infarct dementia. Dementia was the operative word which brought such despair to the three generations involved.

Having cared for both grandmothers who were demented due to strokes and having assisted Mother with my father's care after he became demented due to a severe brain injury (suffered in an auto accident), I thought that I was prepared for anything. After all, we, in my family, took whatever was handed to us and overcame it. We, especially myself, were tough. It never occurred to me that there was a situation in which nothing I could do would help. I was the strong one, the upright post that others leaned upon. I could be super-whatever-was-needed. I had yet to learn the fact that super-whatevers are fictitious characters. I had yet to learn that the only thing I had to hold me up was the super God who had created us, loved us, and stood waiting to care for us.

For me, it was months before healing tears began to flow. I began to clench my jaw, put my shoulder to the wheel, keep my chin up, disguise my fear, and determine not to let this get me down. I constantly reminded myself of our old family physician from west Tennessee, who told me that he had seen three generations of my family through devastating situations that would put an average person down, but that we always got up to fight again. I didn't need to know that. I needed permission to grieve, to become angry, to give up. I needed for there to be some way in which I could say "I can't."

I only knew at this time that faith in God was all I had to hold on to. I had yet to discover that His grace was more important than my faith. I had not yet learned that He would share my burden, lighten my load, restore my soul. The weight of the world had suddenly descended on my shoulders and it was mine alone to bear.

I needed help to adjust, but I ran directly away from help rather than accepting the help offered by friends. I studied all the books, viewed all the videos, tried all the "home remedies"; I worked on memory exercises with Mother. I went straight to work then directly home to care for her. I allowed myself no respite, no rest, no ease. I did everything the hard way, as if I believed that hard work would somehow give better results than accepting help and using labor-saving shortcuts.

I believed deep down that I must have done something terribly wrong for God to have punished me in this way. I never dared express this feeling to anyone for fear that they would agree with me, which would make me feel still worse.

However, life went on. I held on to my faith in God's infinite goodness and believed that He would somehow change the situation. I had not yet learned to lean on Him or to accept the freely given gift of grace sufficient to my needs.

Chapter 2

Caring for Your Loved One—Legally

While we were dealing with the many changes in Mother's behavior, my daughter-in-law was working at Duke University's Geriatric Evaluation and Treatment Clinic and suggested that we have her evaluated there. Mother refused. Eventually my son told her that he had made an appointment for her and she would go if he had to physically carry her.

Although she did not then have enough symptoms to warrant any changes in her treatment or lifestyle, we were encouraged by her physician to have a power of attorney drawn up in the event of her later disability. This we did. I cannot stress too much the necessity for this step when the process of aging begins, even if there are no symptoms at all of approaching dementia. The same legal documents may be needed in the event of sudden illness, accident, or surgery.

I also want to stress here the importance of discussing the wishes of each family member for drawing up living wills and health care powers of attorney. Some family members may have an almost superstitious fear of putting their wishes on paper. If so, make certain that you know their wishes and have them verbalize these wishes to their physician. My mother always refused to put anything in writing. When we had suggested for many years that she make a will and a living will her response was always that I would know what she wanted and that I was the only one to be considered since I was an only child. She could not be convinced that state laws varied and that I might not necessarily be given the direction of either her estate or her health care. In addition to the practical necessities of the mentioned documents, there is an emotional security for all family members in not having to make difficult decisions in the midst of an emergency. In fact, when I realized the complications inherent in dementing illnesses, I immediately drew up all these documents relating to my own health as well, so that my sons would not be faced with tough decisions at a time when emotions are running high.

In the event that more than one person may be involved in the care of one who is demented, having open discussions and legal documents in place prior to need may avoid family quarrels later. Taking advice from a specialist in geriatric medicine, as we did, can smooth out many rough spots.

Some of the most frustrating, yet the most humorous, incidents of our journey have come as a part of caring for Mother's legal affairs. We were some months, if not years, into her illness before I realized that she was not competent to handle her business affairs. I took over her bills, taxes, and so on at that time, and for the first year there weren't too many problems. She had only been paying the minimum payment due on any of her revolving charge accounts, so I began to make larger payments. Her taxes were not difficult at that time either. The complications arose later when she had to be placed in a skilled nursing facility in an emergency situation. Since her income was not quite large enough to cover the cost of her stay there, Medicaid stepped in, which meant that she was only allowed to keep a small portion (the amount varies from state to state) of her income. That small portion would not stretch to cover the payments on her charge accounts and I began to make the payments from my income. This was brought to an abrupt halt when I became disabled and was forced to live on my savings for the nine months before my own Social Security pension was granted. To my surprise, creditors were totally unsympathetic and unwilling to work with me in any way to make arrangements to complete paying the amount owed. In addition to daily threatening letters, I received daily telephone calls, which were even more threatening. I eventually was able to stop the telephone calls but continued receiving threatening letters.

My mother had no assets that could be sold to pay off her debts, and even if she had, I had been informed by the state that whatever assets were left upon her death were to be taken to reimburse the state for the Medicaid funds expended. I was quite amused during one of the many telephone conversations with one of the major credit card companies when the gentleman calling offered to change my mother's account to my name and issue me new cards with a fairly substantial credit limit above the amount still owed on my mother's account. I told him that made me worry about the future of his company. After all our conversations regarding my lack of ability to pay my mother's debts from my own funds he was offering a credit line to someone who was unemployed, disabled, and had no source of income or hope of any in the near future.

The next legal problem arose when I was informed by my mother's caseworker that I should have the income tax that was withheld from her monthly pension stopped. Upon telephoning the appropriate governmental body in Baltimore, I was told that my mother had been deceased since December 1974. After strenuously insisting that she had been very much alive fifteen minutes earlier when I had left the nursing home, and thereafter going through two or three levels of staff members, I spoke to the department head and told him my story, relating how each department had told me the same thing for two hours. I assured him as well that my mother was not only alive but was physically quite healthy. I also informed him that it was my father who had died in December 1974. When he continued to insist that it was my mother who was deceased, I became exasperated enough to ask him to send me a copy of her death certificate, so that I could take her out of the nursing home and have her buried. He, loyal civil servant that he was, was not amused. Nor was I by that time.

The following year I had the identical problem when I brought her home to live with me and needed to have her income tax withholding reinstated. After clawing my way up the bureaucratic ladder, I eventually reached the same gentleman. Early in our conversation I reminded him that I had yet to receive the letter certifying her death upon which he said, "Oh! I remember you." I remarked that I had thought he would. This time was different, though. I had learned to laugh at the absurd aspects of Mother's legal affairs.

These are only two of the many situations I have faced in handling my mother's business affairs. All appears to be on track now, but I never know when that may change. It is at times like these when God gives me the gift of humor to get me through the anger and frustration. If you are the family member designated to handle the legal aspects of your loved one's care, expect to be faced with problems of bureaucracy at all levels. And learn to laugh early. Contact with an attorney who is experienced in Alzheimer's disease or any form of senile dementia is much to be desired at the very beginning of your walk.

Chapter 3

Surviving the Diagnosis

For God has not given us the Spirit of Fear, but of Power, and of Love, and of a Sound Mind.

2 Timothy 1:7 (KJV)

It may seem that this chapter should precede the one before, however, getting the legal affairs out of the way at the earliest possible moment will leave you with less to deal with as your deeper emotions become involved. Additionally, doing something practical helps ground us as we begin to let the realization sink in that we are in a life-changing situation. To be informed that a loved one is afflicted with a dementing illness is to be brought up short in whatever plans we had for our lives. Our lives will be changed in ways that we cannot begin to imagine at the beginning.

If you are reading this book it is more than likely that you are expecting or have recently received the diagnosis you have been fearing for some time. No matter how well you may think you have prepared, hearing the physician verbalize the diagnosis and what you may expect is still a shock. You will realize that you have been hoping against all hope for a miracle pill, treatment, diet, surgery, or anything that will postpone, if not cure, this condition.

In brief, and depending on what stage the disease has reached, you may expect progressive memory loss; personality changes;

loss of ability to perform tasks such as bathing, dressing, and so on; and loss of appetite or its reverse—eating everything in sight including house plants and cleaning supplies. Some patients may become violent, others may become more soft and accommodating. Some may lose their socialization skills, others remember exactly which fork to use at a formal dinner while forgetting their name. Some may sleep all the time, others may suffer from acute sleep disturbances. Some may wander away if not watched carefully while others are afraid to leave their room.

No patient will exhibit all the possible combinations of symptoms, but each will undergo changes that will require mental and emotional adjustment on the part of the caregiver. Even harder to accommodate is the fact that several different behaviors may manifest on the same day. You may find yourself dealing with a totally different person in the afternoon than the one you dressed that morning.

The earlier you are able to turn to God with your hurts, fears, and other concerns, the earlier He will be able to help. It was only when I was indeed able to cast *all* my cares on Him that He was able to respond to me and to take the weight of my burden. This is, perhaps, the most difficult task you will face during the course of the disease. Each of us has developed our own habits of independence. We feel that we can handle all our problems alone, and, if we can't, something must be wrong with us.

I am reminded of a card I gave to a friend who had become disabled that read "Faith isn't faith until it's all you have to hold on to." How easily I gave her the card and how difficult I found it to do when it was my turn.

My oldest son was an extremely independent child. When I attempted to help him with something I thought was too difficult he would stamp his foot and shout, "I do it my own sef (sic)." This was my attitude toward caring for my mother. I felt that if I only read enough books, studied enough scholarly literature on the subject, and tried enough techniques *I could fix her.* Probably many of you will begin with that same outlook.

However, whether you hear the words "Alzheimer's disease" or "multi-infarct dementia" it still remains cruelly true that this person you love will be dying slowly before your eyes. The body you have known for so long will eventually house a personality you don't recognize. You will watch as loss of memory, dignity, emotional control, and behaviors change this person beyond all recognition. Even having known that the time was coming, it is a major shock the first time your loved one forgets who you are. As both a loving daughter and a loving mother I found it impossible to believe that she didn't recognize me. I felt that even if my mind failed, my body would somehow have retained the memory of having carried and given birth to my children. I was so hurt and angry that it took several weeks to come to terms with this stage of degeneration. After seven years of living with this situation, there are still days when I feel a stab of hurt when she asks, "Who are you?"

All of this sounds extremely frightening. If your loved one has received such a diagnosis you will already be frightened, confused, and angry. It is OK, normal, to be frightened. It is at this time that God's words about the spirit of fear find a home in your spirit, not just your memory. Each time I approached a new facet of the disease I repeated this scripture over and over to myself until it became such a part of me that it has carried over into every aspect of my life, including my own disability. In fact, when Hurricane Fran roared over Durham in 1996, God had so filled me with His assurances of watchcare and protection that, while others listened and worried, I slept through all but five minutes of the storm. In that five minutes I moved from my bed immediately under a window to a couch away from windows, murmured a prayer, and went back to sleep.

When my mother's physician said, "I'm not saying it's Alzheimer's but . . . I would recommend that you get in touch with the Alzheimer's support group," I felt that I would faint. I squared my jaw, maintained my dignity (I hope), and attempted to be a cool, logical businesswoman. I don't recall asking anything else sensible. Knowing my behavior patterns it is quite likely that I smiled at him, thanked him, and left him with the impression that I wore a "Great Stone Face" and was totally emotionless and uncaring. I know that we didn't stop for lunch on our way home as we usually did. In fact, I have no memory of driving home at all. I know that after I had given Mother lunch at home I went to my room, better known as "the black hole" both because it had no windows and because it was the room where I went to brood when in deepest pain, and sat staring at the wall and remembering everything I had ever heard or read about Alzheimer's. I formed a mental image of the disease as being like a giant amoeba sitting on top of the brain extending pseudopods and nibbling little portions of brain cells daily. In plain language—I was crushed and frightened beyond sanity. When I returned to work that afternoon and had cried on the shoulder of one of my co-workers, I could not concentrate on my work as usual. I continued to visualize this disease from a science fiction point of view as "The Amoeba That Ate the Brain," something like the movie *The Tomato That Ate Manhattan, The Blob,* or other such pictures. Later I imagined the disease as being a demon from Hell who had sunk his talons into her brain and was laughing at me as he destroyed more and more. He seemed to be saying "no hope, no hope, no hope." Even my prayers during this period reflect my lack of preparation. I never prayed for strength, wisdom, or knowledge. I prayed "make it go away," "make her better," "let me die." At times I wasn't sure if I was praying for my death or hers. After having been the caregiver for my two grandmothers and having assisted with my father's care, I think I must have felt that I had been given more than a fair portion of the bad side of life. My own depression added to my feeling of helplessness and fear of the future. I'm very thankful that I had already begun therapy and gone through the beginning stages of establishing a therapeutic relationship with my doctor. If I had not had this place where I felt safe to be open about my fears, sadness, and yes, even anger, I'm not sure just what would have happened. I needed someone to listen who was not judgmental, did not chirp in a bright and shiny voice that I should "hang on," and gave me the help I needed to stay fixed in the here and now. Thoughts of suicide were very seductive at that time.

Depression is very common in families of loved ones with Alzheimer's disease. In fact, depression is common among Alzheimer's patients as well. You may need your geriatric specialist to recommend someone for your loved one to see. Certainly you should see someone yourself. Depending upon the depth of your needs, you may choose from support groups, caring friends, or pastoral counseling, all the way to full-fledged psychotherapy.

During this period of adjustment I was blessed with the daily companionship of a dear friend and sister in the Lord who was going through the same trials with an aunt in the same condition. We know now that God looked ahead and saw our need for each other long years before we were acquainted. Even now, when her aunt has gone home to be with the Lord, and my mother fails to recognize our relationship so that I have effectively lost my mother, I thank God daily that I have this, the sister I needed and still do. Our love and friendship for each other has only strengthened as we have "rounded up the prayer posse" over the years to pray for all kinds of situations.

Back to practicalities. You must plan, from the very beginning, for some type of respite care as well. You will not be able to handle twenty-four-hour responsibility without a break. Again, this is not what I did, but what I should have done. It was almost seven years until I took a three-day weekend and visited my son in Florida. During those years I became ill myself, but continued to attempt to push past my illness so that I could be the "be all, know all, do all" regarding my mother's care. When I finally took my mini-vacation and arrived in Florida, my son asked me what I would like to do. My answer was that I wanted to spend the whole time without making a decision of any kind. He was to make all the decisions and I was simply along for the ride. Such sweet relief I could not have imagined. I spent hours in his back-yard playing "fetch" with his dog. He took me in his boat down the Intracoastal Waterway to St. Augustine for lunch and I sat, fascinated, as the salt spray and rain fell upon my upturned face. I watched herons along the shore and gazed with delight at the lighthouse as we arrived in St. Augustine. Every morning I went onto his patio and rejoiced that I had no medicine to administer, no breakfast to prepare, no bath to give, no dressing to do, no decisions to make. I rested. This is as necessary to the primary caregiver as food, shelter, and clothing. I was able to return to my duties with a fresh outlook, even though I had only been gone three days.

In the interim between totally getting away there are always periods in the day when you can enjoy respite of some kind. These will be discussed later in Chapter 12, "Taking Care of Yourself."

Chapter 4

Choices: Stage One

But if any provide not for his own, and specially for those of his own house, he hath denied the faith, and is worse than an infidel.

I Timothy 5:8 (KJV)

Unless you have not received the diagnosis until your loved one is far too demented to participate in his or her own choices, you will need to have a family meeting to discuss plans for care. If you have siblings, you may want to make decisions about who will handle which part of the care needed. Each family member, including the patient, will need to consider his or her own family duties and work situation. The patient may need to make a decision or have one made for him or her as to retaining the old family home or moving into a smaller, more easily kept home. This will be especially needed if it is felt that your loved one will be able to remain at home and handle most of his or her own care for some period yet. You will also need to address at some point the issue of whether it is safe for your loved one to continue to drive.

Driving becomes quite an emotional subject when dealing with the elderly, demented or not. In general they view any attempt to stop their driving as an assault on their independence and it is supremely important, in their eyes, that they remain independent.

Due to poor eyesight, my mother had not been able to drive for several years prior to becoming ill, but it had taken a near-fatal accident to convince her that she couldn't see well enough to drive. My father never consented to stop driving, so we were forced to become quite assertive and sell his car and make sure we kept our own car keys away from him.

You will also need, at this time, to make sure that you do not make promises or decisions out of pity, pain, or grief. I, never realizing what it would mean, had made a promise to my mother over twenty years ago that I would never place her in a nursing home. As her disease progressed and I knew that placement would become necessary fairly soon, I felt "locked in" by this promise and thus postponed decisions about placement until it was an emergency situation.

This promise was also the greatest source of my guilt feelings while trying to make decisions regarding placement. I cried out to one of my dearest friends that Mother had said that she wanted to die in the house where we lived. My friend, in her wisdom, said, "But she did. The person you are dealing with isn't Grandma anymore." When Mother's physician said the same thing the very next day, I felt that I had received direction and confirmation from God that I was making the right decision. Even then I was too weak to proceed with planning. I visited one nursing home and came away so upset that I dropped the whole idea until, at last, the emergency situation arose making it an immediate necessity that she be placed.

It is at the early stage of a disease that you should begin to look at nursing care options. You will need to visit several nursing homes and begin to form choices early. If you choose to have your loved one's care provided by a home nursing agency you will need to investigate the agencies available. It is always a good idea to talk with others in your position for references or warnings about certain homes or agencies. Check with the Better Business Bureau to find out if there have been any complaints against the agency and check with social workers for the same information.

If your choice is to take your parent into your home and provide care yourself, you will need to consider just how far you will be able to go with this option. You will need to consider other family members under your roof, your work situation, your own health, emergency options, respite care, etc.

I was eventually forced to place my mother in a nursing care facility due to my work schedule and my inability to find a reliable home nursing companion. I was only able to bring her home, which was my option of choice, when my own health failed to the point that I could no longer go outside my home to work. The possibility still exists that my health will fail still more or conversely that I will get well and be able to return to work and I may be forced into placing her again. If this becomes necessary, I will be better able to deal with it knowing that it is in God's timing and His will since I have given the problem to Him.

When and where to place your loved one will be discussed in Chapter 14, with some practical tips for rating nursing care facilities.

It is at this stage when the choices you make may be very difficult moral decisions. Do you have the right to place your parent's care ahead of your spouse and your children? Conversely, do you have the right to place your home situation ahead of the best possible care for the one who cared for you when you were helpless? Can you place your career on hold for the years necessary to care for your loved one? What if you can't re-enter your career after a ten-to-twenty-year hiatus? Will this loss of income place the burden for your care on your children? Have you reached the stage of faith in which you can fully depend on God to supply your needs and be comfortable and secure in that dependence?

There is no one right answer. Prayerfully consider all the choices, get advice from experts, from those who have gone through the situation before you. Discuss it honestly with your family and ask for their feelings on the matter.

Whatever your decision may be, do not allow it to be influenced by feelings of guilt. We are not all able to handle the emotional baggage of caring for a demented person. We are not all financially able to put our careers on hold. We cannot all disregard our other duties. A balanced approach is all that God expects of you, and He will give you guidance when you truly turn to Him for help.

Chapter 5

Giving Up

Come unto me, all ye that labour and are heavy laden, and I will give you rest. Take my yoke upon you, and learn of me; for I am meek and lowly in heart: and ye shall find rest unto your souls. For my yoke is easy, and my burden is light.

Matthew 11:28-30 (KJV)

This chapter begins, once more, with things I should have done, not things I did. After the diagnosis I immediately read every book and magazine article in Durham County, North Carolina, dealing with senile dementia in all its forms. I found books that were quite good at describing the various stages of the diseases and what could be expected. I found a pitiful dearth of material written for the caregiver who was muddling through on her own as I was. Especially lacking was anything that could give me the inner resources I needed to cope with this tragedy. I had expected, as an only child, that I might someday need to wait on my mother after a heart attack, a stroke, or cancer. I never expected to care for a stranger in my mother's body. My emotional coping skills were at ground zero when the bomb fell. My only advice to the reader is to accept this period as part of your adjustment to the disease process. It will never become easy to give up, but you will find it much easier when you give it all up to the One who created your loved one.

In this early stage you will find yourself attempting every suggestion written, even those, or maybe especially those, which make no logical sense, while attempting to deal with emotions you never expected. We went through vitamin therapy, crossword puzzles, memorizing poems, separating buttons by color, literally everything I had heard of. Each stretch of the imagination seemed to frustrate my mother more. Some Alzheimer's patients deal quite well being in structured activity programs. Some, as my mother, become much more agitated when faced with problems they can't solve. These will bring on behaviors that seem totally insane to the caregiver, but very sensible to the patient.

My mother went through one stage, lasting about a month, of folding paper. She took apart the daily newspaper and folded each sheet into a two-by-two-inch square making it almost impossible to reassemble and read. She went through another stage, shorter lived, of cutting up clothing. I was forced to hide all sharp objects. Mother didn't deal well with guests so I stopped inviting people into my home. She is home once again and I am once again not encouraging visitors other than old friends. She deals well with old friends but is extremely anxious with strangers. She doesn't remember anyone's name but does seem to have a vague memory of the faces. She always tells her visitors that she loves them. This strikes me particularly as a blessing for she and I were never able to say "I love you" to each other until she became ill. This was classified as "silly," so simply was not done.

Antianxiety medication seemed to make her more anxious and to disturb her sleep pattern even more. We discontinued this fairly early and attempted other coping techniques.

Eventually she went into a period of refusing to eat or drink. I chased her around the house attempting to get her to take a bite of yogurt or a sip of Ensure. She lost weight, a great deal of it, and became dehydrated. I again failed to realize that she could not deal with my schedule. I was attempting to feed her in the period prior to my leaving for work, during my lunch hour, and at our usual dinner time in the evening. I did not realize that she could no longer eat at that speed. It was beyond my comprehension at that stage that her ability to chew and to swallow had been affected by the disease.

By this time, I had started utilizing a home health aide to sit with her for part of the day. This wasn't satisfactory at all since we were never notified if the aide couldn't come. My neighbor and another dear sister in the Lord watched and prayed then called me at work when the aide didn't appear.

It was at this time that Mother began to stand on the front porch all day, becoming more and more sunburned and dehydrated. She never attempted to wander away but we were not sure just when that might happen. Again, my sister in the Lord prayed so long and so fervently for an angel to stand with her and prevent her from wandering that she almost felt that she could see him.

I had "babyproofed" the house so that she would be safe when I was not there. In addition, she was fearful and anxiety-ridden if left alone at all at night. I still did not feel secure enough to leave her alone to attend support group meetings, which I so desperately needed. When she was seemingly at the point of death, it was necessary to place her in a nursing home. There she received some of the care she needed, but so much was lacking that I basically had to carry on two jobs at once.

Every morning I went to the nursing home to feed her, back to the office to work, lunch at the nursing home to feed her, back to the office, back to the nursing home for dinner and bedtime preparations. They "forgot" to feed her, change her, turn her. During this period I became acquainted with family members who came to the nursing home daily before breakfast and stayed with their loved one until after bedtime. I didn't wonder why, I knew that they could not feel secure about their loved one's care unless they were present. Complaints made to the administrator or the nursing director reached deaf ears. Ditto the medical director. Turnover in the administrative staff was so high that I was very rarely able to communicate with the same person twice. The particular problem immediately faced might be solved, but a larger one would emerge.

When my mother was placed in the Special Care unit, her care improved greatly. However, there was no restraint on violent patients and I watched those around her being injured. I worried still more.

The time arrived when I came home one evening broken and devastated. I dropped to the floor in the living room and started to weep. I asked God, "What else can I do? I'm at the end of my strength and my ideas. *Help!*"

I couldn't cope with the silence, so I got up to put a Gaither videotape into the VCR, not noticing which it was. Back to my position weeping on the floor—then I heard, I'm not sure yet who was singing, but the song was, "Give Up and Let Jesus Take Over." It was at that moment that the answer came. I had prayed over and over for a miracle, for a healing, sometimes even for her death or mine, but had never turned my worries or fears over to the One who was most prepared to care for her. I learned that I could not give up every care at once and that this giving up would be a continuing process throughout the remainder of her life. However, I was able, one day at a time, to give up small bits of worries. It was then that I seemed to hear Jesus say, "Don't sweat the small stuff."

I didn't worry about her missing dentures; I gave them up. I didn't worry about lost laundry; I gave it up. Daily I learned that there was more "small stuff" than I had realized.

At the same time I was becoming physically disabled myself. Eventually the time came when I could no longer go outside my home to work, so I decided to bring my mother home and care for her myself. There was little required for her care that I didn't have to do for myself. Fortunately she was not a "wanderer." Even here I have had to learn to give up. I think I expected her to be so happy to be home that she wouldn't step on my one frazzled nerve that day. On those days when she is particularly agitated I don't attempt to work with her on memory functions or any other areas of interest. We just take the day off.

Bringing my mother home has provided me an opportunity afforded to few in this day's frenzied world. I have had the opportunity to work one-on-one with her. Her illness continues to grow progressively worse but some facets of her personality have been retained and through focusing on what she can do rather than what she can't, I feel that I am having some small success in holding her semigrounded in the here and now. By watching and listening acutely I am able to recognize signals that she can't verbalize. I have learned that in conversing with her she becomes "overloaded" and breaks the conversation by saying that she must go to the bathroom.

I have learned what situations she can tolerate and those that confuse her unbearably. It is very much like caring for a two-year-old except that she cannot be intellectually challenged without confusion. I have learned that giving her too many choices is extremely disturbing to her. I no longer ask her what she would like to wear but make sure that the clothing I put on her is her favorite color. I no longer ask her what she would like to eat. I serve her plate and tell her what each item is. Again, I make sure that I serve foods she particularly likes. After she has eaten all she will of her meal I put out snack foods and let her make a choice between them for her "treat." When I take her out to eat as a treat I order for her rather than confuse her with choices. Her only complaint is that all servings are too large. She can consume a large meal but only if it is given to her in small amounts.

In the difficult situations, which once caused me great frustration, bathing, eating complete meals at once, and so on, I have "learned to lean." I have "given up." Jesus always takes over at the point of my need and gives me just the ideas I need to get past the situation troubling me. In the event when there is no answer, that part of her mental function is finished, I give it to Jesus and

He gives me rest for my soul. She has forgotten God. She doesn't understand when I discuss Him with her but I continue to do so and to reassure her that even if her memory of Him has failed that He will never forget her.

All of this having been said, and being true, some days are so frustrating for both of us that we must simply stay in different parts of the house. Feelings arise, "hot" buttons are pushed, situations deteriorate that cannot be lived through until we have worked through our emotions. These are the days when I find myself rushing out the door, grabbing a rake, a hoe, anything, and working frantically on the yard while wishing to put my fist through the nearest wall. This is when "one day at a time" won't work. I must pray for the strength to make it through one minute at a time. These are the days when I not only pray for her but with her. Sometimes she will sit quietly during the prayer, sometimes she gets up and walks away, but I feel that at the deepest level she realizes that I am asking God to help us get through a difficult time and she is glad.

"Giving up" in no way means to imply that I have been able, or would expect to be able, to sit back and have God drop by K-Mart to pick up a package of socks or a nightie for Mother. Giving up involves giving the worries and cares to God, which serves my energy for the practical details I can handle, although even here God moves in my behalf. Many times when I am wondering just how I will be able to get out to take care of an errand, a friend "just happens" to call to say, "I'm going to be out and about; could I pick up something for you?" I see God's hand there as well as in the spiritual battles He has fought for me.

My response to these movings of God in the everyday-ness of my life has been a difficult lesson to learn but one that all of us, as caregivers, need to learn early and well. We have to shed that pride bump; we must stop saying "I do it my own sef"; we learn instead to say "Thank you, Lord" and "Thank you, friend."

In the seven years of our walk through this valley so far I have been forced over and over to mentally bow my head and say, "Yes, Mom," when my friends Jean or Priscilla chastise me for trying to be Superwoman. They're right, and they love me enough to tell me to sit down and let someone else help. I urge the reader to learn from my difficult experience in this area that we are not expected to be more than we can be. We are only expected to do what God wills to the best of our ability. He will take over from there.

Chapter 6

Anger: When "Nasty" Creeps into Your Life

Be ye angry and sin not; let not the sun go down on your wrath.

Ephesians 4:26 (KJV)

Anger is one of the most violent of the emotional storms you will be facing during the care of your demented loved one. You will find yourself feeling angry and betrayed by your loved one for having developed and given in to this entrapping disease. You will find yourself angry with God for allowing it to happen. You will become angry with family members and friends who are not as interested as you feel they should be. You will be angry with the medical establishment because they have so little help to offer you. You will be angry with careless motorists on the highway, slow checkout clerks in the supermarket—angry, angry, *angry.* Most of all you will feel angry at yourself because you can do no more than you are doing and because you have been angry with all the above. These feelings of anger toward others can be transformed into guilt and self-condemnation and even more isolation. This isolation will stimulate more anger and more guilt in a circle that can become never ending unless you learn to deal with this most powerful emotion. This anger and guilt cycle will drain you of more and more emotional energy until you feel so drained that your chosen task is even more difficult.

I should know all the above. I must be the world's greatest expert on having and attempting to repress these emotions. I've experienced anger so heated and tormenting that it seemed that my rage must boil over into violent action. I've actually gone out with an ax and cut trees to vent this rage. After the anger I've felt so guilty that I wished to scourge myself with a whip. After this guilt I've been so angry with myself for feeling guilty that my whole physical being is in turmoil. I develop migraines, I have esophageal spasms, I feel so dirty and unworthy that I have not handled myself better and maintained better control. I never give myself any "brownie points" because I don't act on my anger. Only guilt. I've had to learn to deal with these feelings in the "school of hard knocks."

A few pointers you need to learn as soon as possible:

1. Anger is an emotion, a feeling—just that. In and of itself it is neutral. It is when we use that emotion destructively against ourselves or others that it becomes something bad and sinful. The first step in learning to deal with this emotion is to forgive yourself. Yes, yourself. *You* are the one pointing the finger of blame at yourself. *You* are the one laying the guilt trip on your-self—not God. In the verse at the beginning of this chapter God doesn't say, "Don't be angry." He says, "When you are angry, don't allow your emotion to cause you to sin."

2. Realize that some anger is justified and that it requires action. Just make sure that your action is in line with God's will for the situation. If you are visiting in a nursing facility and discover that your loved one who can't feed himself has not been fed or has not had enough time spent feeding him, anger and concern is perfectly normal and right. This calls for action, and, if expressed constructively, your anger can improve the lot of more than one resident. If you see your loved one being treated as a nonperson and mocked or mistreated, this calls for action. You may see strangers looking and laughing or pointing toward your loved one in stores, restaurants, etc. You will become angry.

In almost every case when this happens it is due to the public having so little understanding of the dementing illnesses. I have continued to take my mother on outings when it is appropriate and safe for her. I urge you to do the same for your loved one. It is best for our loved ones to remain a part of normal society for as long as possible. Focus on your loved one—not the disease, and do not be dissuaded by embarrassment or anger. There is no shame in being ill.

3. Forgive God. Now *that's* a scary remark, but just think about it for a moment. He's God; He doesn't need your forgiveness—but you need His and you need to forgive Him to get your relationship back on track. Stop blaming Him for something He didn't do. No matter what your denominational creed may be, the fact remains that God did not give your loved one this fearful disease. Our present state of technology has caused our life span to outstrip our quality of life. Even though we give up the situation to His care, we do not stop our fight against it. He expects us to fight—in the laboratories, in the home, in the hospitals. He doesn't expect us to lie down and play dead and say, "It's just God's will and we must be submissive." No, He expects us to fight with all we have then ask Him for the strength to come back and fight another day. Never lose sight, however, of the fact that we are fighting the *disease,* not the patient. We must learn to recognize early that our loved one is not defined by the disease he or she carries. I suffer from chronic depression, this does not define me as a person. I am *not* a depressive; I am a person with a disease called depression. My mother's Alzheimer's disease is not *who* she is. Regardless of what is going on with her memory or her behavior, she is still my mother. It is she who taught me to read; it is she who once spent hours combing through my long, tangled hair and grumbling at the chore while she refused to cut it. Dementia changes none of that.

4. Forgive your friends and family. Everyone is not emotionally equipped to handle dementing illnesses. We may find friends

and family drifting away. We must remember that our friends, too, have their own problems to face. They cannot be available to us each time we need them. If you are one of those who is motivated by service, remember that we don't all have the same motivations. You may have been of service to a friend who had illness in the family, then had that friend fail to respond in like manner. You may have made an "open-ended" offer to help others in your social circle, your church, your club, but have no one call or send a card when you need it. Again, those who have not faced a dementing illness have no knowledge of the kind of help you may need and may avoid you because they don't know how to help. You will begin by feeling hurt, then anger will slip in, followed by guilt, and your isolation becomes deeper. I feel this isolation today especially. Why today? It's Sunday, a beautiful sunshiny day. Neighbors, back from church are working on their lawns or taking drives in the country. Some are shopping. Some are napping. And some—some are visiting friends. I have been very alone this week. I have raked leaves and spoken briefly to the neighbor across the street. I have spoken to a stranger at the library, I have spoken to two friends on the telephone. I have spoken to my mother who doesn't know what we're discussing. I feel that I am slowly disappearing. My mother is dying and I am becoming a shadow who will have no substance once her life is over. Dementia can be very frightening to those not having had experience with it. My own personal opinion is that watching a patient with Alzheimer's disease may remind many of their own helplessness to avoid that very fate. I'm certain that those of us who are the children of Alzheimer's patients feel that fear. Sometimes I watch my mother and wonder, "Am I watching myself ten years from now?" It is in this area that support groups, which will be discussed in a later chapter, become so vitally important. Anger can be defused and a certain amount of the isolation overcome through these groups.

5. Forgive your loved one. It may seem totally outrageous that we would be angry with the patient, but it happens. As the disease progresses and our burden becomes heavier, we find ourselves becoming angry, not only for the present-day problems but for issues not addressed years ago. We ask ourselves, "Why should I have to spend my life providing emotional support when he or she didn't provide it for me?" We may say, "How could you have done this to me? Why did you refuse to stay active and alert after you retired? Why did you let yourself go?" We must realize that whatever issues were not settled before that it's too late to settle them now. We must remember that our loved ones did not choose this disease. We must forgive them even though they've done nothing wrong. Our emotions keep insisting that it's their fault. We must, one step at a time, work through this feeling until forgiveness comes, over and over and over. I see spouses, primarily women, who are angry because, "He would never let me handle any of the business; now I don't know how." Again, don't sweat the small stuff. If we don't have children who can help us a myriad of experts out there can either teach us or do our taxes for us. I never learned to buy a car. My husband always took care of that. Now, while I don't suffer from AD, I still don't know how to buy a car. I call my son on the phone and say, "I need a car." He chooses what I need, brings car and papers to be signed and I don't have to worry. If you don't have children you may have a good friend. Someone is always there to help.

Anger cannot be dispensed by following the few tips above. It will recur time after time in situation after situation. Realize this in advance and lighten up on yourself. Don't try to repress the feeling. Instead find creative ways to deal with it.

One of the situations that angers me most is having someone—anyone—treat my mother as a nonperson simply because she suffers from dementia. This situation I address immediately. I insist that she be treated with the dignity due any human being no matter how bizarre her behavior. Yes, there is behavior that brings forth laughter, but I do not tolerate mockery.

I do breathing exercises for stress management for my own illnesses. These may help some caregivers deal with anger. They don't help me with it. My own particular remedy, if there is no one available with whom I feel free to talk, is to sit at my computer and write out just exactly how I'm feeling. I don't worry at that time about grammar or syntax. I just feel through my fingers onto the screen before me. Some days there are multiple pages of these writings. After the situation causing the anger is over I can keep my writings for my journal or erase them just as I please. Each person will have to find his or her own method, but finding one is essential. Anger will kill if not dealt with.

I have been reminded again and again, in traveling through the anger portion of giving care, of one phrase in the physicians' Hippocratic Oath—"Above all, do no harm." I have made every effort, no matter how angry, to do no harm to my loved one, to myself, to my friends and family, or to my relationship with God.

One other thing we must remember when we become angry with our loved one: we probably became angry prior to his or her illness as well. Our present anger is no better or worse than before. It is a normal human emotion, felt in all families. The difference lies in the fact that we have to develop new coping techniques when the loved one is no longer able to disagree constructively.

Even as I write this volume and have been practicing coping techniques for venting anger, there are times when I "lose it." Last night was such a night. I am disabled, suffering from chronic unremitting irritable bowel disease. The disease is never under control but is worse when I catch a "bug" and am weaker than normal. I was extremely ill last night and my mother was quite distraught. She has always become very fearful when I'm ill, even prior to her illness. It was as if she always knew that I had to be well and strong to care for her. She refused to eat at dinner-time. She refused to go to bed at bedtime. She refused to take her shoes off when she finally went to bed. She sat on the side of the bed and picked the decorative needlework out of the bedspread. Each time I arose and escorted her back to bed she became more frustrated and I became more angry. I considered going out and sitting on my stump but felt too ill. My fever was over 102° F.

At midnight Mother was standing in the kitchen screeching, "I want something to eat. Do you want me to starve?!?"

I arose again, began preparing her a small meal and scolding her at the same time for keeping me awake. This time the quarrel escalated to something on the order of a nuclear bomb blast and we were off into a "I did and then you did and you never when I wanted" type fight. I did note in some small part of my mind that long lost memories seemed to be regained with the stimulus of extreme anger. I realized all the time, of course, that this was achieving nothing of value, that it was only bringing on an anger, guilt, anger, guilt circle and that I would have to work through all these feelings when I was calmer. Nevertheless, I was still out of control at that time. The quarrel ended with my grabbing a blanket and pillow and announcing dramatically that I was going to sleep in the car. She went to her room, came back with all her jewelry on and announced that she was moving out. We settled that one by my going into my bedroom, slamming the door and locking it and dissolving into tears. She sat at the kitchen table the remainder of the night waiting for someone to come get her so that she could move out. This morning she is not speaking to me even though she doesn't remember why. I'm feeling a weight of guilt much heavier than the situation requires. I remember that this is exactly like the quarrels we had when I was a teenager, which always resulted in her not speaking to me for some days and my asking forgiveness over and over. In our anger we both reverted to a time when we each knew who we were and what we wanted. In a way it was like "going home," even though unpleasantly. I know that I will apologize for becoming angry with her and that she will respond by refusing to speak to me today. Maybe, in some way, that is the comfort zone we look for when remembrance of the hopelessness of the disease overtakes us.

For whatever reason we descended to this level I realize that I am now the adult in this situation. It is up to me to control my actions and hurtful words. I promise myself again that I will be more careful, that I will defuse my own anger before responding to her but I know that times will come when I will still "lose it." I'm so thankful that God is a forgiving God as well as a loving one. I'm so thankful that I can turn to Him for help in controlling my actions and for comfort when I fail.

Five days after this quarrel we are still not on good terms with each other. I do not feel able to take her out for a drive. She has no concern or no ability to feel concern for my health and rages that I'm depriving her of any pleasure in her life. I refuse to answer her in the same frame of reference but attempt to soothe her out-of-control emotions while I exist on a diet of Tums. I rake the same part of the yard for the fifth or sixth time. I transplant bushes that could wait until I feel better. I scrub the floor on my hands and knees—nothing helps. She tells me she is moving out. I tell her I'll buy her a one-way ticket just as soon as she decides where to go. She gets sick. I feel guilty.

I pray again. "Oh, God, just help me to get through this one minute in time, just one minute at a time." He does. He sends a robin to the tree over my kitchen window to sing "pretty, pretty, pretty." He sends the stray cat, Mush-Mush, who has adopted me and lives under my shed to the door to "meow" for my attention.

So we go through that day, one minute at a time, and at last it's bedtime and I can have at least two hours rest. The indoor cats curl around me on my bed and purr as they rub their heads against my chin. If things seem really bad to them, Widget dashes to the door and spits, sputters, and swears at Mush-Mush through the screen to make me laugh, while Tat looks on with great disdain and says to me, in "Catonese," "Aren't the children silly?"

I sigh with relief, arise to check on Mother one more time, then come back and squeeze between the cats who have taken their half of the bed exactly in the middle, and say, "Thank you, Lord."

We have to realize also, that anger on the part of our loved ones is many times a disguise for the fears they are unable to express. The connections in the brain which once made communication possible have become tangled and the words pouring out may have no relation to the thought behind.

At one time I had a transient ischemic attack (TIA) and upon reaching the Emergency Room was unable to tell the attendants that I had a tremendous headache. When they asked where my pain was I kept repeating, "chest, chest, chest." This inability to communicate was so frightening to me, even though short-lived, that I cannot bear to think of how it must feel to live every day in this condition. Unless it happens to be one of the isolated instances when I "lose it," I try to find the emotional root of my mother's anger. She may be in pain, she may be lonely, she may be confused about who and where she is, she may not like the clothes I put on her today—any of these can bring on fits of anger and agitation, which she will express by saying, "You just don't like me."

At these times I can only look to my Father and ask for wisdom to discern which emotion I need to address. He has been so faithful in directing my thoughts that I am overwhelmed at His great love and mercy to one person when He has a whole world to care for.

Chapter 7

Agitation, Sleep Disturbances, and Other Disasters

Your loved one may make it all the way through the disease without developing any behavior problems. The likelihood, however, is that you will find yourself facing some of the behavior problems discussed here and will be as clueless as I was as to how to react. I have titled these behaviors "disasters" because they seem to occupy an inordinate amount of our attention and energy. You may find yourself wishing, as I did, for a tornado, a hurricane, an earthquake or any other natural disaster simply because it would hit and be over—not a nightmare that seems to promise it will never end.

Sleep disturbance has been one of my mother's primary problems from the onset of the disease, so we'll start there. About one year after she was diagnosed, Mother began to pace the floor all night. Prior to this, and even prior to her diagnosis, she had begun to be extremely easily awakened. It was my habit, prior to her symptomology, to set my alarm clock an hour early and have my morning devotions before anyone else was awake. Before we even knew she was ill, she began to intrude on this quiet time by coming into my bedroom and chatting until I could not concentrate. I reminded her over and over that this was my prayer and Bible study period.

Her only reply, and that in a hurt tone, was, "Well, if you're bored with a lonely old woman I'll go away. Maybe someone, somewhere will want me."

Of course this set off the guilt trip reaction in me and I assured her that I was not bored and that I definitely wanted her. I began to set my alarm for 2:00 a.m. and put it under my pillow so that it wouldn't awaken her through the wall. This really didn't do much for my prayer life. I found myself dropping off to sleep during my devotions. Without the time I normally spent with Him, I felt in a desert far away from God.

Another nocturnal entertainment for her (still before diagnosis) was what my son and I referred to as "playing in her closet" all night, every night. She would take all the clothes off the hangers and rearrange them. Since her closet wall backed on my bedroom wall it was impossible for me to sleep while this was going on.

As the disease progressed and she was diagnosed, she began simply "rambling" all night. At the time we lived in a two-story house and I was afraid of her falling during these rambles. Each time I heard her get up I arose and put her back to bed. I asked her physician for assistance and he attempted to help; however, she had adverse reactions to all antianxiety medication and sedatives. She became still more agitated and rambled all the more. Eventually I wedged myself in her doorway against a pillow and snatched a few winks while I was in a position to stop her before she got out of the room.

I never asked how the nursing staff at the nursing care facility where she was placed for a little over a year kept her in bed. Maybe because personnel were always awake they just let her ramble. I never saw any mention of sedation on her chart and I did review it frequently. At any time that I inquired about the behavior patterns I had tried to cope with at home, I was assured that "she was doing fine." But "fine" in a nursing home with around-the-clock supervision is not necessarily "fine" at home. The less she slept, the less I slept. At the time I only brought her home for day visits so I couldn't see for myself what went on there at night.

After bringing her home to live I soon found that she still followed the same patterns of sleep disturbance. I knew that sedation was not the answer, but asked her doctor's permission to try two ounces of wine at bedtime. I tried this remedy and it did seem to help—for approximately a week. After that her old pattern emerged again so I gave up the wine.

After "babyproofing" the house I tried just staying in bed and letting her ramble to her heart's content. Then she began to sit on the couch in the living room and drop off to sleep in such a position that she could hardly move when she awakened. I solved that particular problem by piling the couches so high with pillows at bedtime that there was no place for her to sit. In response, she got up, came to my room, and awakened me. Sometimes she only wants to have a conversation, sometimes she asks me to come sleep with her because she is lonely, and sometimes she seems satisfied just to know that I am awake and "on the job." Now, if she merely "plays in her closet" (which used to disturb me so) or comes to sit at the kitchen table and stare into space, I turn over and go back to sleep. (We have moved to a small house with no steps.)

If Mother has been so persistent in her disturbances that I have missed sleep altogether, I follow the pattern I followed when I had a sick infant in the early days of motherhood—when Mother dozes during the day I take a nap also. If it seems that a pattern of daytime sleep is emerging, I begin waking her each time she drops off for a nap, asking her to move to another place to sit. By the time Mother has moved, she is wide awake again. I try to keep her that way until a normal bedtime. However, she always suffers an adverse reaction if I attempt to keep her up too late at night. If she stays up later than 9:00 p.m., she doesn't sleep at all.

Monitor your loved one's sleep carefully. Mother's sleep disturbances must be monitored and dealt with constantly for both our sakes. What will I do if her pattern changes again? I don't know. But I do know that in some way God will provide either the strength to go through it or the idea I need to overcome it.

During some of the earlier stages of the disease Mother's agitation was at a much higher level than it is now. Looking back, I believe that she must have been worrying about losing her memories. She didn't realize that she was ill but did realize that she was "different" somehow. She looked for people long dead, she looked for home, and she looked for familiar clothing. Home especially seems to be a time and place indescribable, some thing in her she knows will never be recovered. She was obviously searching for that place in her mind where she would once again feel normal and in control.

At present she is calmer most of the time. She occasionally begins to search for someone or some place once familiar. On these days she is, what she calls "very upset." She asks what I have done with her daughter Beth. She shrieks at me that I am keeping her husband away from her. She thinks that a ride in the car will take her to find the place where she will feel comfortable. If at all possible I take her in the car and we ride, sometimes in the country, sometimes in the city, until she becomes calm again and asks to be taken home.

Another disaster is bath time. Mother becomes highly agitated, and from discussions with others, I find that this is fairly common among patients with dementia, even in the nursing homes. In the earlier stages of her disease I was stronger and able to physically lift her into the tub even with her kicking and screaming. I am no longer able to do so. After bringing her from the nursing home to live with me I attempted to bathe her in the handicapped shower stall, but after being knocked down and bruised, I gave that problem up also. I now give her a sponge bath—the kind she was accustomed to in her childhood.

I no longer insist that she sit and eat a complete meal at once. I place her food before her and leave it. She eats a few bites, wanders away, and then comes back many times before it is finished. I tease her that she eats one meal a day—all day long.

So much of this is "the small stuff" that I have learned to give it up along with all the other parts of the disease I can't change.

Each one of you will be dealing with behavior changes in your loved one. They may not be the same changes I have dealt with. Some may be much more difficult; some may be much easier. Once again, the answer is in learning to lean on God for wisdom and strength. We must always remember that love is the key, and we are dealing with a person we love rather than a disease we hate.

I have learned to look for the emotions behind the behavior. I know when my mother becomes extremely agitated that she is probably more confused that day. I attempt to be calm and reassuring. I tell her she's doing "just fine." I tell her over and over that she is my mother and I love her. I remind her that I will take care of her so she doesn't have to worry. I tell her that God is taking care of both of us.

I have no idea what goes on in the mind of an Alzheimer's patient, but I have a suspicion that somewhere deep inside is a tiny core of the original person. This tiny core may be capable of feeling trapped by the inability to communicate or to control the behavior of the body.

Sometimes her behavior reminds me of a funny occurrence in the emergency room of the hospital where I worked. It was July 4 and celebrations were taking place all over town. Even though it was a "dry" county, liquor was available in any quantity desired if you knew the right folks. Two automobile accident victims were brought into the emergency room, neither hurt seriously but both quite inebriated. As the physician began to clean and dress their wounds he asked the first patient who had been driving. The patient replied that he didn't know.

The physician asked the second patient who had been driving and his reply has always stayed fixed in my memory: "Well, Doc, it were like this; I was sittin' behind the wheel but they wasn't nobody drivin'."

I envision my mother's mind as this automobile, with her body sitting behind the wheel as it goes careening into disaster, and the tiny core of herself that remains knows that no one is driving. It must be terrifying.

Chapter 8

Dialogue with Dementia: Communication Problems

For the first few years of my mother's progressive descent into dementia, I fought desperately to believe and to convince others that somewhere inside her was still the seed of her own personality, and that if I worked patiently enough and kept myself informed on the issues, I could help her return to a state of relative normalcy.

After many years of trial and error with daily work on memory functions I wonder if I have fought in vain, for our daily dialogue is such that I wonder if it is she with whom I am speaking, or her disease. I desperately want to believe that locked up in her brain somewhere is a key that would unlock her memories if we could only find it. Just as desperately I doubt it and am afraid that I am caring for her disease instead of her person.

This is a sample of our dialogue on a "normal" day, beginning at 7:00 a.m.:

Me: Good morning, Mother. How do you feel this morning?

Mother: Good morning. Who are you?

Me: I'm your daughter, Beth.

Mother: Are you sure?

Me: That's what you've always told me. Do you remember when you gave birth to me in Westport?

Mother: I don't believe I do. Who was your mother?

Me: You are. You're my mother and I'm your daughter, Beth.

Mother: Well, if you're sure I guess that's all right. Do you think it is?

Me: Do I think that what is all right?

Mother: That you're my daughter.

Me: Of course.

Mother: I just didn't know what to do.

Me: Just sit down at your place and take your medicine. I'll have your breakfast ready in a few minutes. (She sits, pulls a worn and frayed picture of President Clinton from her purse and smiles at it.)

Mother: Now that's my purse.

Me: Yes, that's your purse. Please take your medicine.

Mother: I just didn't know what to do. Am I all right?

Me: You're fine. Now put the two little white pills in your mouth and take a sip of your juice to swallow them.

Mother: Is that all right?

Me: Yes, that's what the doctor said to do.

Mother: I don't have a doctor. What did Beth say?

Me: (Giving up the struggle to let her know who I am.) Beth said you should take your medicine.

Mother: I don't want but a little bit.

Me: OK, but swallow your pills.

Mother: What about this cup?

Me: Swallow that too.

Mother: I just didn't know what to do. Would it be all right if I went into that closet and peed?

Me: Of course. Don't forget to flush and wash your hands.

Mother: I just didn't know what to do. Am I all right?

Me: You're fine. Go pee then come back and eat your breakfast.

Mother: I'm not very hungry.

Me: You have to eat anyway. Go back and wash your hands.

Mother: What's this?

Me: That's scrambled egg, that's ham, that's toast, that's coffee.

Mother: I can't eat that much.

Me: O.K. Just eat what you can.

Mother: I want something out of that bag. (Cheese curls)

Me: After you eat your breakfast.

Mother: (Screeching angrily) I told you I'm not very hungry! Get out of here and leave me alone!

Me: I'm going outside to drink my chocolate. I'll come back in when you calm down.

Mother: You calm down yourself. Go find Beth. I want her.

Me: (After going out onto back stoop and drinking chocolate) After your breakfast we're going to wash your hair and give you a bath.

Mother: I don't need a bath. I just had one this morning.

Me: No you didn't. You had one day before yesterday and you *must* have one today.

Mother: Why?

Me: You smell bad.

(She takes approximately two hours to eat breakfast, thereby postponing bath time.)

Mother: I just didn't know what to do.

Me: Now take off your glasses, your jewelry and your blouse; I'm ready to wash your hair.

Mother: Wash *my* hair?

Me: Yes.

Mother: Why? I just washed it this morning.

Me: No you didn't. Now come over to the sink. We *must* wash your hair today; it smells like perspiration.

Mother: (Speaking to her picture of President Clinton) *She* says my hair smells bad. I wonder what *she* did with Beth.

Me: Come along now. The longer we put it off the more you'll dread it.

We begin to shampoo her hair:

Mother: Oh! I'm hurting. Stop, Stop!

Me: What hurts?

Mother: I don't know; the water, it's too wet.

Me: It may be uncomfortable but it can't hurt you.

Mother: Did you lose it?

Me: Lose what?

Mother: I don't know. I just didn't know what to do.

Me: Now stand up so I can dry your hair. Now take off your bra.

Mother: I won't have anything on.

Me: I can't bathe you with your clothes on.

Mother: I just didn't know what to do. Do you think I'm all right? Will Beth be back soon?

Me: I'm sure she'll be back soon. In the meantime let's finish your bath.

Mother: I just didn't know what to do. I just didn't know what to do.

Me: I'll tell you what to do. That way you won't get confused. Will that be OK?

Mother: Are you helping me?

Me: Yes.

Mother: Will you go find him?

Me: Find who?

Mother: My boy. The one I live with.

Me: Are you talking about Jimmy?

Mother: Yes I want to go home with him.

Me: You don't live with Jimmy, Mother. You live here with me.

Mother: Who are you?

Me: Pay attention now. I'm your daughter, Beth. You're my mother, Velma. We live together and I take care of you. Do you think you can remember that much?

Mother: Am I all right?

Me: You're fine—now tell me who I am.

Mother: (She looks intently at me) You're my cousin.

Me: No. Guess again.

Mother: You're not my mother are you?

Me: Never mind. At any rate you know that I take care of you.

Mother: And you are so nice to me.

Me: Thank you. Now we've finished your bath, how about going into the living room and resting on the couch for a while.

Mother: I sure do feel bad.

Me: Where do you hurt?

Mother: I don't know. I want to go somewhere in a car.

Me: Later today we'll go to the little store and buy milk.

Mother: Are you sure?

Me: Almost.

Mother: Are you from Huntingdon?

Me: Almost twenty-five years ago, yes.

Mother: Who was your mother?

Me: I don't think you would remember her.

Mother: Can I go in that room and look out the window?

Me: Certainly. You can go anywhere you like.

Mother: Can I sit down here at the table?

Me: Of course.

I continue with washing dishes, preparing lunch and dinner and cleaning the house as she sits at the table and stares into space.

Mother: Do you know where Beth is?

Me: She's probably outside working in her flower bed. Did you want me to get her for you or is there something I could do?

Mother: Go get Beth.

I go outside, walk around the house, smoke a cigarette, blow smoke out my ears, talk to the stray cats, then return to the kitchen.

Me: Did you want me, Mother?

Mother: Are you Beth?

Me: I sure am.

Mother: I'm so glad you're back. I was scared you were lost. Can we go somewhere in your car?

The foregoing conversation (?) to the uninitiated seems totally meaningless. To those of us who have—through long and painful necessity—learned to speak the language of dementia several things are clear from this conversation:

1. She is more confused than usual today. Recall the number of times she says that she "just didn't know what to do."
2. She has some realization of her confusion and it is frightening. See how she asks, "Am I all right?"
3. She sees me as a nurse or caretaker today rather than as a family member. She is asking for my son so that she can feel secure. This is usually brought on by bath time (which she hates) or any change in her routine.
4. When she is most confused she loses her appetite. She must be soothed before she can eat. Notice that I left the room until she was able to become calm again.

On days when she doesn't recognize me she is much more concerned about herself. She asks repeatedly, "Am I all right?" Attempts to convince her of my identity as her daughter only bring on quarrels. She must recognize me herself for us to have any meaningful conversation.

A dialogue such as this continues throughout the day until bedtime. I close myself in my bedroom for twenty minutes twice a day and do relaxation exercises and arise strengthened to continue the dialogue. I feel pity, anger, frustration, and fear. I know she must feel most of the same emotions. I try to answer patiently and when I find that I can't, I leave the house and walk around the yard until I calm down again. I know that I want to scream "Just give me ten minutes of silence. Can't you entertain yourself for ten minutes?" I know she can't. I treasure the time after she has gone to bed and resent it if the telephone disturbs my silent time. I tiptoe around the house in the morning hoping she will sleep late. I drop something in the kitchen and the dialogue begins again.

Not all days will our dialogue be as harmless as this. On some days anger and frustration boil over and the dialogue, stimulated in some way by anger, becomes more rational even though hurtful and disturbing. For some reason extreme anger brings back my mother's memories and her old personality to the forefront for the period of time while she is angry. I wish we could bottle the rational part of her anger while defusing the emotion and give it to her in small doses on days when she doesn't remember anything.

Most of us who provide the actual hands-on care for our demented loved one know that we spend a great deal of time in "fantasyland." We have learned the hard way that attempting to convince our patient that he or she is irrational only brings on more confusion. Sometimes, after having a particularly difficult day, I awake the next morning to the sound of my mother rambling through the house. I keep my eyes closed and wish myself into a fantasyland of my own. I dream that I'm in a cool, old-style Florida home on the banks of the Pithalachascotee River in Port Richey. A waiter, looking vaguely like Fernando Lamas, comes into my room with a tray of breakfast and a lovely rose in a crystal vase. He opens my drapes and I look out on the sun-dappled waters as they flow into the Gulf of Mexico and I rest as I eat an elegantly prepared meal that someone else cooked.

That's about as long as my trip to fantasyland lasts. Widget comes to awaken me and I pretend to sleep a few more minutes. At last I open my eyes. I look toward my eagle plaque on the opposite wall, ask for God's help for strength for the day, shove my feet into well-worn slippers and my body into a bedraggled robe and proceed to the kitchen for another day:

Me: Good morning, Mother. How are you this morning?

Mother: Who are you?

Chapter 9

Individual Differences

For as the body is one, and hath many members, and all the members of that one body, being many, are one body: so also is Christ.

1 Corinthians 12:12 (KJV)

Just as each of us is born with and continues to develop different personality traits, patients with senile dementia will exhibit different symptoms. Do not expect your loved one to develop all the symptoms or stages of the disease you have studied. By the same token, do not be surprised or afraid if he or she shows symptoms you have never heard of.

Yes, there will be tremendous personality changes. The person inhabiting the body you have known and loved may bear very little resemblance to the person you have always known. For your own peace of mind and reduction of stress accept each new personality and make friends with it. Do not attempt to hold onto the old personality. This will be frustrating in the extreme both to you and your loved one. Realize too that this is not a case of multiple personality disorder. The personality changes you see are caused by an organic disability of the neurotransmitters to perform their job. This disease cannot be helped by psychotherapy. If, at some future date, it is discovered that dysfunctional thinking has laid fertile ground for the devastating attacks of the plaques and tangles on the brain cells, psychotherapy would need to be begun much, much earlier.

You may have learned to accept and live with the new personality only to find a momentary flashback of the old personality appearing at the most unexpected times.

In addition, personality traits may be so deeply ingrained that they will remain dominant even in dementing diseases.

My mother always dealt with uncomfortable feelings or events by "tuning them out." She still does, but phrases it as "I just don't remember." She has learned to verbalize that feeling. She tells me that she "just can't bear to hear about anything unpleasant." In some way she has achieved an understanding of her emotions that she never recognized prior to her illness. She always told me that when I was faced with some unpleasantness that I should "just put it out of my mind." If, when I receive letters from old friends back in Tennessee telling of the ill health or death of someone we once knew, she leaves the room in the midst of my reading the letter. Later she has no memory of having received the letter at all. Her memory for unpleasantness is just as selective as it was in her early life.

Mother still remembers the daughter she knew as "Beth" who stood in her place when she was afraid, misunderstood, etc. She does not recognize the person who insists that she be bathed, medicated, put to bed at night. She has designated that persona as *"she who must be obeyed."* Mother doesn't like *she*. Quite often she awakens me in the middle of the night demanding to know what I've done with her daughter Beth. Arguing with her that "Beth" and *"she"* are one and the same is fruitless. I have learned to tell her that Beth will be back soon or that I will go and get Beth for her if her need is urgent. She is a great admirer of President Clinton and carries his picture in her purse. I hear her telling him of the injustices perpetrated by *"she."* Sometimes I laugh, sometimes I cry, depending on my own state of emotional health.

I learned early that memory exercises requiring judgment or manual dexterity were terribly confusing and frustrating to her.

Now, if she is able, we sit and look at family picture albums and I ask her to identify the photos. I tell her stories from my childhood and later life involving her and she laughs with me but doesn't realize that I am discussing us.

I ask her if she remembers a certain old friend. Sometimes she does, sometimes not. I don't insist; I don't push. Today she asks me how my father is; tomorrow she will tell me that he has been dead a long time. Sometimes she thinks that I was married to him. She must be imagining that I am a younger her.

She checks herself frequently saying, "This is my purse; these are my shoes; this is my necklace; these are my glasses" and ends by asking me, "Am I all right?" I assure her that she is fine.

She has developed a fascination for trees. Each time we go outside she asks me to, "Look at those trees. See how tall they are." As we drive down the highway she keeps telling me to look at the trees.

Each patient with a dementing illness will develop characteristics particular to his own personality or stage of the illness. We cannot look at another person's loved one and see what we may expect of our own.

We deal with the personalities we are given, we accept them, and we make friends with them. I have had to realize that "Mother" is no longer with me but I still remind her daily that she is my mother and I love her. Whatever personality she wears that day still seems to appreciate and be reassured by being told of my love.

Some days it seems that it all becomes too much and I look at her and realize that "Mother" is gone and will never return. A few years ago I lay in a hospital room of my own with IV medications running and listened to the sounds of hospital life around me. I realized finally that I was listening for the sound of my mother's footsteps coming down the hall to visit me. I faced the fact that I would never hear that sound again, no matter how sick I was or how much comfort I needed. Now I feel bereft and rootless in a world where a disease has stolen my connection to my roots. It is then that I realize that my Father, God the Almighty, has never changed, never gone away, and is my connection to all my yesterdays and all my tomorrows. It is then that He brings me comfort above and beyond anything I had dared to dream of.

Chapter 10

Fears, Phobias, Fantasies, and Other Foibles

But the fruit of the Spirit is love, joy, peace, longsuffering, gentleness, goodness, faith, meekness, temperance: against which there is no law.

Galatians 5:22-23 (KJV)

I am a self-admitted phobic. If I become demented and exhibit hallucinatory tendencies I'm positive I will see spiders everywhere and no one will be able to safely drive across a bridge with me in the car.

Those of us who are parents will remember the days of monsters under the bed or in the closet and the very necessary soothing of these fears.

Having dealt with fears, phobias, etc., with both my grandmothers and both parents in their dementias, I realize just how much time and energy, not to mention of patience, can be involved with this facet of care. The patience needed will be the "longsuffering" spoken of in the opening Scripture passage. This aspect of care may involve more patience than any of the behavior changes or emotions other than anger.

There are no pat answers for any of these behaviors. What works for one patient may not work at all for another. The method you used this morning may not work this afternoon. It is an ongoing process requiring great attention to judging just what the emotional need of the moment is and how it can best be handled.

My first experience of the turmoil brought about by such behaviors was when one of my grandmothers stripped off all her clothes and ran up the street naked. This grandmother had been extremely modest so there was absolutely no relationship to any former behavior. As with her daughter, my mother, antianxiety medication made her worse. After trial after trial the method that finally worked was to sew all the openings on her clothing together and split the clothing down the back. Each morning when dressing her I then stitched the back of her clothing closed and she couldn't get undressed without aid.

This was my first experience with caring for a demented loved one and absolutely every technique was a matter of trial and error. I'm surprised she didn't have a stroke simply from frustration with my bumbling attempts to handle her disease. I had absolutely no idea of the emotional aspects of care and thus remained so focused on the merely physical that during her remaining life with me she must have felt emotionally deprived. I really can't speak to any fears she might have had. I never thought to wonder about *why,* I only worked on stopping the behavior.

By the time she had gone home to be with the Lord and my other grandmother began to develop strange behavior patterns, I had realized that there must be something going on in the brain to cause these actions. I had begun to wonder about the *why* of it. In studying abnormal behavior, the only literature available to me was texts on abnormal psychology. Remember, these were the "good old days" when the diagnosis was always "hardening of the arteries." Of course most texts on abnormal psychology dealt in depth with psychiatric therapies rather than senile dementia, but there was enough there to make me sure that something was behind the bizarre behavior patterns. When this grandmother became demented she would be quite paranoid and imagine that there were intruders who planned to attack and kill her. Knowing, by this time, that attempts to argue her out of her fantasy would be fruitless, I simply entered the fantasy with her and assured her that I would protect her by killing the intruders. With this assurance, both she and I would be able to sleep. Notice that there is no seeming relationship between the behavior patterns of the two grandmothers. The marker which shows that something like the same process was at work is the fact that both of them exhibited behavior which was totally alien to their prior personalities.

My father was a different matter entirely. He and my mother had supported and had in their home all their married life a combination of his parents, her brothers and sisters, and assorted aunts and uncles who needed a place to stay. I was their only child but we had a full house all my life. My father had dedicated me to the Lord at birth to go as a foreign missionary. He had been extremely disappointed by my decision to marry and raise a family instead. When he became ill much of his thought was still involved with the foreign mission field. In addition to this, my mother and I had determined that it was too difficult for her to care for the large two-story house on five acres of land where they had been living since their marriage. So the home was sold and they moved into a smaller house with a smaller yard near my home so that my family was more readily available to help. Daddy was in a strange place with memories only of his work with the mission board.

I had taken the night shift at the hospital where I worked since this always meant either my husband or I were at home with the children and that I was available to help Mother in the daytime with Daddy's care.

He was always searching for "home." I spent endless days driving him to all the places where he had ever lived, searching for "home." I did not know at that time that home is not a place on a map, but a time, an area of familiarity, somewhere you feel "normal." In addition to searching for home he imagined he was on the mission field. When storms arose he would watch the trees

bowing and swaying in the wind and rave about "heathens danc-
ing on his lawn." No one could convince him that what he saw
was trees. Of course I couldn't stop the action of the trees and
drawing the drapes had no effect. I could only attempt to reassure
him that "they would stop soon." Because of my father's wishes
for my life and the fact that I let him know that I did not choose
to spend my life according to his wishes, we had a very poor
relationship. He was so disappointed in me that he could never
see any good in anything else I might do. I was so resentful of his
disapproval that I had as little concern for his feelings prior to his
illness as he did mine. When he became ill I felt such guilt that I
had never let him know that I really loved him but just couldn't
live his lifestyle. Because of this guilt perhaps I watched his
emotional problems more closely than those of my grandmothers. I spent more time trying to address his emotional needs.
I'm not sure if my being motivated by guilt played a role or not
but I seemed to be less successful in finding the emotion behind
the action than I had been with his mother. At last, I was with him
one afternoon so that my mother could get out and run some
errands. He was attempting to escape. He would now be designated as "a wanderer." I was refusing to let him out the door. I
had just come off a fourteen-day stint at work and was too exhausted to take him out for a drive.

As I was standing before him at the door, firmly refusing to let
him out, all his rage at me overflowed and he shouted over and
over, "I just hate you; you've never done anything right."

I'm sure that my reaction was partly due to my own anger and
partly due to my exhaustion, but instead of shouting back I found
myself saying, quietly and calmly, "I don't particularly like you
either, but you are the only Daddy I have, I'm the only child you
have, and I guess we're stuck with each other."

For some strange reason a peace descended upon both of us
now that it had all been said. He lived another eighteen months
and we never had another harsh word between us. He was much

more receptive to my work with him and my anger had disappeared. He still went into rages but they were "generic," never personalized. I often heard him in his room shouting, "God damn you, God." He would have cut off his own tongue before saying those words prior to becoming ill. I always felt that a tiny part of the real Daddy was coming out at those times and that he was angry with God for allowing this awful disease to take him. I knew that God understood and loved him just the same.

On the day he died I had visited him in the hospital where he had just had surgery. His dementia was completely cleared for those two hours and, while not discussing anything of any particular substance, we held each other's hand and were at peace for the first time in my memory. I always felt that God had given us particular grace that day. That years of pain were washed away in the looks and soft words exchanged during that time. I have forever been grateful for that day.

Now I am going through the same process for the fourth time. Mother has lived longer with her dementia than any of my other family members. Part of my being able to work with her emotionally has been because we were much closer all my life than I was to the others and so I knew her better. Part has been due to the increase in information about the dementing illnesses and a great deal has been due to learning to lean on God for the answers or the wisdom to know when to give up.

There are still times when I am overwhelmed by what I consider bizarre behavior, but I can generally work it out given time.

One night recently we had been under severe weather watches for most of the afternoon. We had been warned and instructed by television personnel who were doing a constant update on the severe weather and I had prepared the only area in our house that could be considered safe at all in the event of a tornado.

I don't really consider myself phobic about tornadoes; however, I have a very healthy respect for this most violent of storms. At last we were warned that a tornado was on the ground in our town and that we should take cover immediately. I took Mother into the closet I had prepared, covered our heads with a quilt, had the area lit with a large flashlight and was holding my mobile phone in my hand. Just as I began to hear the roar of approaching high winds, Mother jerked away from me and attempted to get out. I was holding her in place, hearing the "freight train" sound growing closer and closer when she became extremely agitated and violent. She attempted to hit me but I managed to drop enough other things to hold her arm away from me. Just as the wind reached its peak, she managed to break my hold on her arm and get out the closet door. Fortunately the storm was not on the ground when it passed over us. Mother was so agitated and so angry that she was uncontrollable. The increased adrenaline seemed to bring her out of her dementia for a short time and she shrieked at me over and over, "I'll take care of myself *my way!*" My one remaining nerve was quite frazzled by this time and I did not attempt to either argue or soothe but went to my room and closed my door to prevent allowing my sharp tongue free rein as I wished to do.

Upon thinking the whole situation over the next day, I remembered that she had always been phobic about closed-in spaces. We had lived in a tornado-prone area as I was growing up and Daddy would go to the storm cellar but Mother would never go or allow me to do so. She always made sure we sat on a featherbed so that lightning wouldn't strike us but "tuned out" the wind. She talked of the possibility of spiders and snakes being in the cellar. I don't have an answer for handling this problem. I can chase away the imaginary people who might be trying to come in, and I can pretend to go get her daughter "Beth" for her when she is confused. I can't protect her from realities such as tornadoes, lightning strikes, etc., when her fear of the protection is greater than fear of the danger. This is one of those situations I must learn to give to God and dismiss from my "worry banks." I must learn to exercise that fruit of the spirit known as "long-suffering" being translated as "patience" when situations arise in which I am helpless.

When she tells me that her friend, President Clinton, is coming to pick her up to take her for a visit to his home, I can convince her either that he has been delayed or that she misunderstood just when he said he might be coming. I cannot convince her to hide in a closet. I cannot convince her that the piece of rope the cat is playing with is a cat toy. To her it looks like a snake, another of her phobias. I take away the rope and give the cat another toy.

Such situations in this aspect of care for demented loved ones have no good answers. Those we learn, with great difficulty, to hand over to a loving God.

In short, in dementing illnesses, just as in the rest of life, there are no pat answers. We don't have solutions for the great big problem—we just have a *great big God* who is able to solve them for us.

Chapter 11

Role Reversal:
Learning to Say "No"

Children, obey your parents in the Lord: for this is right.

Ephesians 6:1 (KJV)

If you, as I, were raised to a habit of strict obedience to your parents' wishes, this is one of the hardest steps to take—the day when you must become the parent of your parent. The obedience habit is so thoroughly ingrained that, except for the rebellious teenage years, you will suffer acutely as you are required to say "no," "you must," "sit down," "stay in bed," etc., to the one who has always said these things to you.

Some days will be so frustrating that you will wish you could spank or send your parent to stand in the corner. Since these are not options open to you, growing a tough inner hide will be necessary.

You will find yourself standing face to face saying, hopefully calmly, "Either you will take your bath or I will bathe you but *you must* have your bath." Or, "You *must* swallow these pills." "No, you *can't* wear that dress; it's mine and you are too large for it."

Successive repetitions will be necessary until you feel you will either scream or run away. Running away is the better option. In my case I take a walk all the way around my yard, or sit on a stump and watch birds until I am calm once again. Then I remember that the verse says "Obey your parents *in the Lord*" and that I will not be violating Scripture to become the parent and care for my loved one as she once did for me. This is the same Lord who commanded us to take care of our families. He expects us to do whatever is necessary to keep our loved ones safe, warm, clothed, fed, etc.

I realize that in this volume I have dealt solely with the emotional reactions of children caring for parents and ignored the fact that many of you are caring for a spouse who is ill. In retrospect, however, I believe that most of the same things apply. I'm sure that the way that we look at the disease, the patient, and the emotions must be different; however, the emotions are the same—just redirected. As children we expect, in the natural course of events, to lose our parents. We expect to care for them during their failing years. When the loved one is a spouse we never quite believe that he or she, the other half of us, will go away from us in such a way that we can no longer relate as husband and wife. It must be a great deal more difficult to see a spouse become a child again; it must hurt differently to become the parent to your spouse. Again, only God can ease these hurts. Only He can share our load; only He can carry us when we are no longer able to walk beneath our burden. And, as I speak frequently of our burdens, let me define the term. For the purpose of this volume I am not referring to the physical care of our loved one—I refer to the emotional burden of living with losing a loved one to dementia. The emotional burden will bring us down without the help of our merciful Father. Practical care of the physical needs of our loved ones can be exhausting; however, playing golf or tennis can be exhausting as well. We can rest from the physical load. We have to learn to give up the emotional load.

The burden of role reversal can be your breaking point on some days. My mother wears the body of the one who always said to me, "You can't go out today; it's raining and you have a cold."

Now, regardless of how ill I am, regardless of circumstances, she seems to crave excursions most on the days when I can hardly hold myself upright, when I have about a tablespoon of gasoline in the car, and my Social Security check isn't due until next week.

The day then consists of her following me around the house shrieking, "I want to go in the car. You take me in the car *now.*"

The little girl still living inside of me just wants to put her in the car and drive her around while the adult, responsible caregiver knows I must say, "No, I'm not able. We'll stay at home today."

If it helps you to visualize your loved one as yourself as a child, and visualize yourself as your parent, go ahead. Caregivers must hold on tenaciously to our grip on reality but we can allow ourselves to slip into our demented loved one's reality for the time necessary to handle whatever situation has arisen.

While sitting with my friend's mother while my friend was in the hospital we "went fishing" each day. We took a walk around the fenced-in yard on our way to the shop where we bought fishing tackle and bait. Then we walked around the same yard until we reached the "creek" and fished for awhile. I was never sure who was playing with whom. Occasionally I saw a certain gleam in her eye that let me know that I didn't have her fooled for a minute. The next moment the gleam would be gone and we would be fishing once again.

In that case also, my friend had been "mother" to her mother for the many years of her Alzheimer's disease.

Times come when you will long to be a child again, just for a few moments, to be able to lay your head in Mother's lap and rest. The burdens of adulthood seem to be heavier each passing day. It is then that we remember that we are children to our heavenly Father. We can lay our heads on His shoulder, feel the support of His everlasting arms and sink into rest.

Chapter 12

Taking Care of Yourself

Six days shalt thou labor, and do all thy work: But the
seventh day is the Sabbath of the Lord thy God: in it thou
shalt not do any work.

Exodus 20:9-10 (KJV)

If you are the primary caregiver, caring partner, or loving
family member with full responsibility for your loved one's care,
it is of supreme importance, and is supremely difficult for you to
take care of yourself. There may be many motivations for your
devoting your whole being to the care of your diseased spouse,
parent, or other family member. However, the fact remains that if
you don't take care of yourself, you can't take care of them.
Service to others may be the motivational gift given to you by
God but you may misinterpret His intentions for your service. He
never told us to serve until we dropped. Even Jesus rested. How
much more can be expected of us who are only human. Guilt
may be another driving force in your serving until you drop.

You may feel, "If I had only . . . fed him differently, given him
X vitamins, stopped his using X chemicals . . . if only, if only, if
only . . ."

No, you did *not* cause this disease, you cannot with any
amount of service change its course, and you cannot cure it.
Dismiss guilt from consideration in planning for your loved
one's care and your own.

You may be driven, not by any hidden motive, but simply because the task seems so overwhelming that the only way to keep up is to keep on keeping on until exhaustion takes over and you are ill yourself. You may become so fixated on the day-to-day physical care that you don't realize what a toll this care is taking on your body, both emotionally and physically. I'm an expert on all the above wrong attitudes. I made all the mistakes. This is a "do as I say, not as I do" chapter. I have learned the hard way that I must take time for myself. I must have rest; I must have recreation; I must have respite. Remember that God gave us the sabbath as a day of rest. Many times we become so preoccupied with mundane worries that we forget that without this time of rest we will fall by the wayside. Earlier in my mother's disease I became so obsessed by making sure that I did everything myself, making sure she had the utmost I could give in time, care, and attention that, knowing full well that I was ill, I didn't go to the doctor until I was so ill I had to be hospitalized. I felt that asking for help, letting someone else take on some of the chores or worry, would be weakness. Again, my toddler's "I do it my own sef." I had a bump of pride growing right along with my responsibility bump.

A few pointers to better health, happiness, and emotional well-being:

1. Plan, from the *very beginning,* with family, friends, etc., some areas in which they can help.

2. Fix firm goals for rest and relaxation for yourself. For some this may mean a trip to Europe; for others it may mean only a walk in the woods or a shopping trip. The point is to fix these goals and keep to them.

3. Make time for yourself to commune with God. Be exceedingly firm in holding to this time. Your relationship with Him is more important than anything else in your life. If you must lock yourself in your bedroom, go sit in the car in the driveway, etc.; keep this time if everything else fails.

4. Accept help when it is offered. I remember well receiving a letter from a dear lady in my church offering to "baby-sit" with my mother so that I could get out. Pride reared its ugly head and said, "I can't possibly keep my house in the pristine condition it would need to be to have an outsider come in to see." I appreciated the gesture and so informed her but refused to accept the help. With 20/20 hindsight I realize that this was plain stupidity.

5. Stand back and look at your whole situation and make decisions about what can be dropped, what changed, and what must be done. You will be surprised at the many things that are not really must do's. Remember that toaster cover you must launder—really, how many pieces of dusty toast have you ever eaten from an uncovered toaster? You may be, as I was, a totally unabashed "granola," believing that each time I used a paper towel I was causing the death of a tree and building a new landfill. You will find it necessary to change some of your very fixed habits. I have had to realize that for the present I do not have either the time or the energy to spare to launder extra towels and napkins. I simply plant an extra tree in my yard to replace the ones I feel I have despoiled.

Each of us has some "pet peeve" that we simply hate to do. Mine was cutting my mother's toenails. I finally realized that it was much more sensible to have it done by a podiatrist and to save my energy for something more important. Don't wait five years to make these choices, as I did.

6. Forget schedules. Breakfast, lunch, and dinner do not absolutely have to be served at 8:00, 12:00, and 6:00. Baths do not absolutely have to be on Mondays, Wednesdays, and Fridays. Unless your loved one is incontinent, those sheets don't have to be laundered until tomorrow.

7. Watch your own diet. It is far too easy to get so busy caring for your loved one that you fail to eat properly. A Ritz cracker and a slice of cheese eaten on the fly does not take the place of fresh vegetables, fruits, and grains.

8. Keep your physician appointments. Don't neglect to tell your physician of any problems you may be having out of fear that he or she may recommend rest or respite for you. If recommended, follow the physician's advice. When I became ill enough to be hospitalized, I insisted that I could not enter the hospital until the next day because I had to make arrangements for someone to check up on Mother in the nursing home and arrange for someone to care for my cats. It never occurred to me that both of these could have been handled from the telephone in my hospital room.

9. Join a support group and attend regularly. Arrangements for someone to care for your loved one during your absence may be difficult, but not impossible. Making new friends who are going through the same problems helps you to feel less isolated and you will learn coping strategies that you will never learn in any other place.

10. Maintain contact with your old friends. Don't wait for them to call you! Some of them may not be able to deal with watching the progression of the dementing illness of your loved one. Some may not understand the seriousness of the matter. Some may simply not want to "bother you" during your difficult times. But you have a telephone. Use it! You need the love and understanding you will receive from those who have been your friends for a long time.

I have also reintroduced letter writing in my household. It's much easier to discuss all the news when you don't have a mental image of dollar signs on your phone bill floating through your mind.

11. Make sure that you get away—completely away—for relaxation occasionally. Realize that you are not the only person in the world who can care for your loved one adequately. If finances are a problem, and they can be, take a day trip but get completely away from your situation. On one occasion I spent the day in the North Carolina Museum of Art in Raleigh. I bought a poster for my grandson, I ate at a restaurant while reading a novel, I

stopped at the airport and watched airplanes take off and land and I sat on a park bench in the sun and daydreamed. When I returned to my situation at home, I found that I was strengthened and ready to take on my chore again. On another occasion I took a day trip with friends to the mountains. I stood on an overlook and looked into the valley at farms, forests, and black Angus cattle. We all daydreamed about moving to the mountains, knowing full well that we couldn't, but it was fun to dream. Back home again, I was relaxed and ready for my life to continue. I did bring enough of the daydream home to inform my friend that if he, in his travels, found a farmer in the mountains who raised black Angus cattle and was looking for a wife to keep me in mind.

12. Take some time for yourself every day. It may only be fifteen minutes here and there, but it is more necessary than you can imagine. For many years my greatest source of relaxation has been gardening. I no longer attempt to tend a large garden but do take some time every day to go outside and rake, dig, plant, or just pick up branches that may have fallen off trees. I may only plant twelve tulip bulbs instead of the quarter-acre I once would have done, but it is still my hobby and my relaxation. My house has been "babyproofed" so that it is safe for me to be outside for this period of rest and relaxation. If you can't get out, at least got into your room and shut the door. Lock it if necessary, and don't feel guilty. You need this time, and your loved one is close enough that nothing can happen in your alone time. The loved one will (I guarantee) still be there when you come out.

13. If you have placed your loved one in a nursing care facility, do not visit every day. Visit frequently enough to be sure that he or she is being well cared for, but do *not* spend all of your free time at the nursing home. Your loved one will adjust much better also if you are not there as frequently. Quite probably the things you will need to do to take care of yourself will not be the things I have done. Your needs may not be the same, your interests

different, however you need to be quite adamant about taking good care of yourself. This is not a selfish, looking out for number one attitude, but a necessity so that you can continue with care for your loved one.

Remember too that by taking care of yourself now you may be saving your children from becoming caregivers later.

Chapter 13

Smoochies, Snugglies, and Other Warm Fuzzies

A great many studies have been conducted showing how interaction with pets is very therapeutic for demented patients. They seem to be able to recognize and receive the acceptance they obtain from animals more easily than from people. In fact, pet therapy has been introduced in many nursing care facilities. Perhaps this is because pets are so very accepting and noncritical.

If, in your case as in mine, your loved one has never and still does not take an interest in animals, it is still important that you realize that you need the love and acceptance provided by your pets.

Loneliness and isolation are two of the emotions you will find most prevalent in your life during the years you are caring for a demented loved one. It is amazing how pets can warm that icy spot in your heart. As I sit here and write, my cat Widget is perched in my lap conversing with me. Occasionally she reaches up and pulls my chin down so we can look each other in the eye and "kisses" me on the end of my nose. If she has detected some depression or sadness, she will leave my lap and become very naughty to distract me. One of her favorite antics is to swing from the ceiling fan or to get herself into a situation that requires my intervention to rescue her.

I'm not sure of the mechanism which causes animals to appear to know just when you need comfort most. My theory, not based on scientific research, is that since animals' survival in the wild is based on their ability to read body language and voice tones, this may be carried over into the domesticated animals.

I have two cats who have provided me with comfort, love, entertainment, and sheer joy. During the earliest stages of my knowledge of my mother's disease, my older cat, Tat, seemed to know exactly when she should come, crawl into my lap, and purr. If I happened to be weeping she licked the tears from my face and laid her head on my shoulder and purred louder.

My younger cat, Widget, is the nurse, caretaker, comedian, etc. Her method of comfort is usually to make me laugh by her wild antics. Sometimes she almost seems human in her understanding. If Mother starts rambling in the night, Widget comes and wakes me. If I am ill, she crawls in bed with me and wakes me just before I have an attack of IBD. Widget seems to take her responsibilities very seriously. If I happen to oversleep and Mother is in the kitchen ready for breakfast, Widget comes to my room, yanks my glasses from my face, and pushes my eyelids open with her paws. She gives me very stern "marching orders" all the time I'm dressing, then escorts me to the kitchen triumphantly showing Mother and Tat that she has succeeded once more in setting our world to rights.

When Widget came to live with us as a very small kitten, she looked like no feline I had ever seen. In fact, everyone who saw her asked, "What is that?" I did not choose Widget from the group of cats I was checking. She climbed my blue jean leg, perched herself on my arm and said, "Let's go home."

After putting her down and lifting a prettier kitten, Widget again climbed my blue jean leg, perched herself on my arm and said, "I said, let's go home! I'm your baby!" When we arrived home she walked into the house—all five inches of her—and surveyed the situation.

Then she went immediately to my mother as though telling me, "I'll take care of this one."

Mother, who was very ill at the time, kept picking Widget up by her tail, swinging her around and throwing her across the room. Widget always came back for more. Eventually she decided that perhaps she should hold on instead of allowing herself to be thrown. This resulted in a long scratch on Mother's arm, which I was forced to explain over and over a few days later when Mother was admitted to the hospital. When asked if I harbored a vicious cat in the home with my Alzheimer's patient, I was forced to say, "No, just a self-protective one." All during the next eighteen months when Mother was in the nursing home, I brought her home to visit and Widget went immediately to her, snuggled beside her, and purred until I took her back. Now that Mother is home again, Widget has resumed her duties as principal nurse so is never seen too far from Mother.

I've also established a bird sanctuary in my back yard. The house I moved into when I realized that neither Mother nor I could handle two stories is backed by a wooded lot with a ravine running through it. I've taken the brush and debris left from Hurricane Fran and created brush piles in which birds and rabbits build their homes. I put out food each morning for the birds and squirrels and watch them from my kitchen window as I wash dishes or prepare meals. Mother can't see well enough to watch the birds, but likes to have me tell her about what kinds I see. She laughs when I tell her how the naughty squirrel hangs by his tail from a limb and eats out of the bird feeder. She laughs when I tell her that our neighbor's cat is lurking, waiting for a bird. The cat knows I don't allow her to kill birds but she lurks just the same, looks at my window to find out if I'm watching, and wanders away in disappointment if she sees me shaking my head. At times when I am particularly blue, I go to the window and take great comfort in watching the birds and animals. I believe God must have placed animals here as a comfort to the hurting as well as a source of nourishment.

In the years since my situation as a shut-in, both from my illness and my mother's, I seem to have developed some type of attraction for stray cats. Maybe they pass the information along that there is always food at the Hall house along with a pat on the head and a scratch behind the ears. They don't all come to live, but do visit consistently. Mush-Mush has decided to live here, but Smut and Ick only visit every week or so. Both Mother and I take pleasure in watching their antics. Again, Mother can't see them but loves to hear about them. She is supremely amused when I go outside to pet them and then am attacked by two jealous house cats when I come back in.

Chapter 14

Choices:
Stage Two: Placement?

If you have chosen to keep your loved one at home in the earlier stages of the disease, the time may come when you will be forced to take a second look at your living arrangements. This may happen through being totally overloaded, your employment, your inability to find proper home care, needs of others in your family, your own health, or the rapid decline of your loved one's situation.

If you have followed earlier recommendations and examined nursing care facilities, made financial arrangements, and prepared for this eventuality, it will be much simpler. I had done some of these things in a rather haphazard manner so that when my situation became an overnight emergency, I was forced to take the only bed open. This is not the most desirable situation.

In addition, if you have emotionally prepared yourself for this time, you will be less stressed and more able to handle the last-minute arrangements. I found myself completely emotionally unprepared. The promise I had made many years before that I would never allow this to happen haunted my every plan or decision.

One night in particular I found myself staring at the front door and thinking that for the rest of my life I would be the only one entering that door who belonged there.

The loneliness was, at that point, almost more than I could bear. It was only much later that I came to realize that each time I entered or departed through that door, Jesus was with me.

I learned that I could sit with Him during those quiet hours and study His word in depth, which I had never had time to do before. I learned that He would guide me in my decision making, and simply spend time just "hanging out" with me when I needed a friend. I began to take long walks through His world, and He walked with me and pointed out the beauty I had not been able to see before because of my worry. He built in me such a confidence that He was always with me, that when Hurricane Fran roared over Durham in 1996, taking homes and lives, I slept.

In my particular case, my mother improved in the nursing home enough that she began to beg to come home. At the same time, my own health was declining and I was facing disability. At the point when I finally accepted that I was no longer able to go outside the home to work, I was faced with another choice about Mother's care. Since she needed no special therapies, I determined that I could bring her home where she would be happier. There was nothing needed for her care that I didn't have to do for myself and it seemed easier to handle this at home rather than visiting her away from home.

Although she was receiving good care, I had a genuine loathing of visiting her in the nursing care facility. This may not be a valid choice for many of you. I was a divorcee, and had no husband to be inconvenienced. My children were all grown and married and living away from home. I was the only one to be considered. I have since wondered what would happen to her if my own health declined to the point that I could no longer care for her. I have, this time, prepared both my mother and myself for that eventuality. God has reminded me that He is still able to care for her even if I am not.

Every day since her homecoming has not been a happy, happy day of sunshine and flowers. Some days both of us are cranky. That's normal too in a family.

Things have gone much better since I've realized that it is hopeless to expect "normal" behavior from a demented person.

The question here is "What *is* normal?" I'm not sure we have succeeded in defining "normal" in the general population, much less among the demented. Realizing that she is acting completely normal for a demented person has freed me from the burden of attempting to change her behavior, which only frustrated us both.

She carries her purse everywhere and every time she stops she retrieves from it a picture of President Clinton cut from a magazine and shows it to people, telling them that he is a dear friend. She reminds me constantly that this is her purse. I think she is probably reminding herself.

She has to have her morning medication explained to her each day. The "magic words" are "because the doctor said so." I have had to develop these magic words because questioning everything I say or do is one of the "hot buttons" from our former life that can upset me terribly. As a child, then a teen, she would ask a question concerning one of my suspected misdeeds. When I gave her the answer she would look at me suspiciously and say, "Are you sure?" I always fiercely resented this reaction. I had never told her an untruth and resented having my word doubted. I still do. She still questions my actions using the same words and look. I have had to give this problem to Jesus more than any other. My own response would be a sarcastic rejoinder.

If the point has been reached in your life where your choice is to place your loved one in a nursing care facility, you will need to establish a few criteria. As you are touring the home, notice the odor. Truly, it is impossible to make a nursing home smell like a bower of roses, but an odor that strikes you as soon as you open the door probably means that the home is understaffed and time is not available to keep the patients clean and dry. Notice the movements of the staff. If they are frantically rushing from one room to another, again, the home is probably understaffed. If they appear to be taking a leisurely stroll visiting with each other, then they are not being attentive to their patients' needs. Take a few minutes to review the material on the bulletin board. Incident reports involving patient accidents are required by law to be posted. If the last incident report goes back several years and there is not an award of some kind offsetting the information, take a closer look. Ask questions. Ask how often incontinent patients are changed, ask about feeding schedules, ask about any particular concern you have about any facet of your loved one's care. If you have more questions than you remember at the time, you may get copies of the state laws regulating nursing homes. Each state has an ombudsman program for nursing home patients. Your loved one's physician may have a social worker on staff or may know of one who is an expert on senior care. Utilize all avenues to obtain the information you need to make an informed decision.

If you have placed your loved one in a nursing care facility and have concerns about his or her care, do not hesitate to express your concern. Talk with the nurses in charge, talk with the social worker, talk with the administrator, and put it in writing.

In addition to the above, ask occasionally to review your loved one's chart. If an incident has occurred involving your loved one and an injury ensued, ask for a copy of the chart immediately.

Remember at all times that you are not locked into this particular situation. If you are unhappy with the facility, continue your search and transfer your loved one when you find a more desirable location.

If Medicaid will be involved as partial payment for your loved one's care, a caseworker will be assigned. It is an unfortunate fact of life that they are not all well versed in the rules and regulations regarding your loved one's assets or income. If you are told something questionable, get it in writing. Again, this was something I failed to do. It is to be hoped that legal matters such as wills, powers of attorney, etc., were handled long before this time.

If not, it is probably too late. However, you may want to check with an attorney. Try to find an attorney with some experience with nursing home cases, Alzheimer's disease, and other dementing illnesses. Remember also that there are separate rules for Social Security pensions, Civil Service, and Railroad Retirement Annuities, and private retirement accounts. Never assume that because you have asked to have your loved one's status changed or reviewed by one body that it will be followed through to all bodies concerned. Again, get it in writing. Some governmental bodies do not accept powers of attorney. You should investigate this early in the disease process. You do not want to be involved in a court-ordered hearing to determine your loved one's competency, which can become an adversarial process, when you only want to do your best for the one you love and care for.

Double-check everything. Remember that God gave you a responsibility and you are expected to live up to it. Remember also that He never gives us more than we can bear. His strength is made perfect in our weakness and He never takes a day off.

To provide maximum care and protection for your loved one, visit the nursing home at unexpected times. Try not to make your visits on a regular schedule. You will be better able to determine the consistency of care when you have seen all shifts in operation.

Treat the nurses and nursing aides kindly. They are performing an overwhelming task with very little reward in the way of pay or praise. If you consistently see something happening that you don't approve of, it is probably a company policy that they are locked into. Work with them to improve conditions. During my mother's stay in the nursing home each situation that worried me was the result of a matter of policy rather than poor nurses or aides. Cooperation between the family and the staff who provide direct care can give relief to a situation that you never anticipated.

Chapter 15

Support Groups

In the earliest stages of your walk through this disease process with your loved one, you may believe that you do not need a support group. After all, you have your own circle of friends, family, etc. You may feel that you are much too busy learning to care for your loved one and continue your usual daily life to spend time with a support group. After all, these groups are for those who can't deal with their problems, aren't they? You are strong. You can learn to handle it alone, can't you? *Not!!*

Unless your circle of friends and family include several members who have walked or are presently walking the same valley, they haven't a clue as to how to begin to help you. You will be the one who must educate them and to learn how to ask for help. You will find that you need information only available through groups of people with the same problem. You will find that sitting for a short time each month with those who have the same troubles and discussing your feelings along with practical tips for dealing with different stages of the disease is the most restful and productive time you spend that month. You will find that this time, indeed, is where you discover your "comfort zone."

I have a problem with shyness and am uncomfortable in a group of strangers, so I put off attending a support group meeting for at least a year. I had always been able to stand before a group of any size and give a speech on any chosen subject, but became tongue-tied when faced with one-on-one conversation in a group of strangers. Not with our family support group. Simply in the process of introducing ourselves at the beginning of the meeting, I found that I was in a group of "friends I hadn't met yet." The newsletter I received whether or not I attended the meetings was worth a fortune to me. I found that this was the place that God showed me that I was not alone. Of course I knew that He was always with me and we communicated many times daily. However, in the support group I was able to see His face and know that He had provided this as a respite for me.

In addition to the emotional support received at these meetings, the practical tips passed on may have life-changing consequences. In our "sharing" sessions, and even in sessions when we have a speaker on a particular topic, someone usually has a question such as, "What do you do when he _____ ?!?" Hands shoot up all over the room and those who have experienced this particular behavior are able to give practical advice and describe techniques that worked for them.

In some cases, AD patients become quite fearful and paranoid and may hallucinate that someone is going to harm them. One of my grandmothers had this particular fear in the days long before we had heard of Alzheimer's or support groups. We, as a family, had attempted every known reassurance to no avail. She still insisted that she saw little men on the bookshelves with knives.

On the theory "if you can't beat them, join them," I entered her fantasy, took my small son's cap pistol and shot the invisible men. After this she was able to go to sleep without fear, knowing that I would shoot any intruders. Was it morally wrong to pretend I saw the men who weren't there? I don't think so. No matter how much I counseled or reassured, she still saw them. I simply enabled her to dispel her fear so she could get much-needed rest.

Little things such as this illustration may seem trivial, but nothing is silly or trivial about a lost night's sleep. There is enough lost sleep and rest for the patient and the caregiver as it is. It is this type of practical help that can only be conveyed in groups of people with like problems. It is "the small stuff" that gets in the way of coming to peace and victory over the despair and defeat the caregiver feels at the beginning of the valley.

If I were forced to rank the importance of various people and disciplines in this walk through the valley it would probably look something like this:

1. Geriatric physician
2. Family and friends
3. Pastor and church groups
4. Family support group
5. Geriatric social worker
6. Respite care workers

The physician is for my loved one with dementia. The rest are to help me be the best caregiver I can be. I don't like the term "caregiver," which seems like a job description, and my care for my mother is a relationship, not a job. However, there are certain things a caregiver needs to know which are not part of the normal education of a daughter.

It has been partly a result of the help I have received through the family support group that I have, at last, learned God's will for me for the rest of my life.

When I became disabled, one of the first questions I asked of God was, "What will I do with the rest of my life?" The answer did not come in a blinding flash of light, nor did He speak to me from a burning bush. The answer came slowly, over a period of years, as I cared for my mother, cared for a friend's mother while my friend was in the hospital, talked with other family members and friends about their experiences with demented relatives, studied the field of senile dementia in depth, and participated in the family support group. I realized that He had been leading me all the way and that I wanted to spend the rest of my life as an advocate for patients with dementia and their families. I cannot do this by going daily to an office and staying at a work station for eight hours. However, I can do it from my home. My computer and my telephone are at the service of those who need them. I can do emergency respite care if the patient is brought into my home. I can write, and by a wise adjustment of my medications, I can go out for a short time, upon occasion, to participate in support group and conferences. I can be a listener when a distracted family member needs to just "vent."

There are so many projects just waiting for someone to begin them that I can't possibly do all I have dreamed of. But nothing is ever accomplished without a dream to begin.

I dream of the day when support groups will be held all over the city, in the affluent district and in the slums. I dream of the day when the government will realize that it would be as cost effective to pay family members a salary to stay home and care for their loved ones rather than place them in nursing homes. I dream of the day when the retired college professor, minister, secretary, or accountant with Alzheimer's will be treated with the same dignity that they were before AD.

I dream of the day when society realizes that warehousing our elderly so that we are not obligated to face our own mortality is not the answer. I dream of the day when we will open our minds and our hearts to receive the gifts that AD patients can bestow. Of course I dream of the day when the disease is conquered, or when its onset can be delayed, but until then I dream of our being so familiar and comfortable with it that we will not react with horror and anger when faced with this diagnosis.

I dream of a day when there will be volunteers from each support group to act as sponsors for new members. These volunteers would be willing to serve as a resource when the new member desperately needs to talk with someone who will understand, volunteers who will be willing to walk through the tough times and help to bear another's burdens during the adjustment period, volunteers who would be willing to be a "voice in the night" when times seem darkest and another's voice is so desperately needed. I dream of the "long-timers" taking the hands of the newly diagnosed patient and family and helping allay their fears of the unknown. In other words, I dream of a time when all God's children realize their responsibility to others in the family of God.

I dream of a brighter tomorrow, which can be achieved only with the help of God.

Chapter 16

Survival Pointers for Everyday Life

In prior chapters we have been dealing, for the most part, with emotional issues. However, dementing illnesses bring on definite physical changes as they progress and focusing only on the mental and emotional changes will not be all you will need to know about or to do.

It is simply a fact that the very everyday-ness of problems brought on by your loved one's dementia may just be the last straw you can bear emotionally. Many of the small things that have made life easier for me have come from people who have traveled this valley before me. The simple acts that relieve us of a portion of our worries leave us able to be more focused on more important issues.

Progressive neurological disorders may bring about physical changes you have never expected. Those I discuss are only a few of the possibilities you may face. Additionally, no one can predict which symptom will strike in which order. If you are caring for your loved one in your home and doing the actual "hands on" care you may be faced with your loved one's (1) loss of ability to walk; (2) loss of ability to sit or stand in one position; (3) loss of ability to feed himself, or to differentiate between food and other substances; (4) incontinence, both urinary and fecal; (5) becoming bedridden; (6) falling due to not realizing that he or she cannot stand. The list of problems goes on and on, but anticipating such problems and preparing for them will help avoid the shock factor and make life easier when and if any of these problems are presented.

I was fortunate in that I was of an age that was taught basic home nursing skills in high school. In addition, I had ten years of hospital experience as a nursing assistant and technician. If you have chosen to keep your loved one at home at all costs, it will be advisable to invest in a home nursing course as early as possible. Such a course may be available at your local community college. If not, contact your county extension service for information on the nearest one available in your vicinity. If you begin to notice that your loved one has developed an unsteady gait, start watching for a good walker advertised for sale in the local newspaper. If you cannot find a used one in good condition, have your loved one's physician write a prescription for one. Medical supply stores will generally do your Medicare billing for you on this purchase. If you wait too long to teach the use of this aid the memory function may be so distorted that he or she may not be able to learn to use it.

For less than $100.00 you will be able to purchase supplies to have on hand "just in case" incontinence happens. I call this my "emergency pack." If incontinence happens, the onset will probably be sudden, and unless you have anticipated it by having a few supplies on hand you may have some of your best furniture ruined—definitely not a happy day.

These should be purchased and put away for future use:

1. Disposable underpads—Very much like disposable diapers but larger
2. One package of disposable diapers in the appropriate size
3. A large wash basin like those used for bed baths in hospitals
4. One bottle of soap specifically for perineal care
5. One box of disposable rubber gloves
6. One box of body powder—preferably nonscented. I use cornstarch directly from the supermarket rather than more expensive, often irritating body powder.

These are simply emergency supplies. If you continue home care, purchasing diapers and underpads in volume is more economical. If you are fortunate enough never to need these items they may be donated to a nursing facility or rest home.

In addition to this list, since my mother is not incontinent all the time I use nondisposable underpads (washable, reusable) on the couches, chairs, and in her bed. They can be whisked off quickly and thrown into the back of a closet if unexpected visitors arrive. If I receive a surprise visit before I have time to remove these pads I simply say nothing about them. I do not know how much my mother understands of what is said around her, but I do know that if she understands at all she would be embarrassed by having her incontinence discussed.

If the choice has to be made, for a short time, I will attempt to preserve her sense of self and dignity at the cost of losing some furnishings.

It is of supreme importance if your loved one is incontinent that you never leave him or her wet or soiled. The skin of the elderly breaks down in such a short time and decubitus ulcers (pressure sores) are very difficult to heal. Make sure that the type of diaper you use is sufficiently porous that air gets through to the skin and leave the diaper off at some time during the day for an hour or so.

I assess my mother's skin condition each day, and if she shows any signs of rough skin, bruising, etc., I take appropriate measures. She has a habit of leaning on one elbow very heavily to help her get up from the bed, chairs, etc. I must watch that elbow very carefully to avoid a pressure sore. I bathe it daily, apply moisturizer and massage it for at least five minutes. All of the supplies you will need for incontinence care or skin care are readily available at medical supply stores and most large drugstores.

It is to be hoped that your loved one will never need to be restrained, however, he or she may reach a stage of not being able to walk but not remembering this, so is in real danger of injury. A relatively simple method of restraint that I have used successfully with one grandmother and my father is to secure a folded sheet, folded about one foot wide, around the patient's chest and chair with large safety pins at the back of the chair. This sheet should be tight enough to be relatively secure but not tight enough to cause difficulty in breathing or circulation. Escaping from restraint and falling is the lesser of two evils since restraints of any kind, unless very carefully applied, can be deadly. Your loved one's physician may prescribe a Posey chest restraint, which is also readily available at medical supply stores but should, under no circumstances, be applied until you have had expert instruction in proper application.

In the event your loved one becomes bedridden, remember that all joint areas will be under pressure on the bed. If left in one position too long pressure sores will develop, normally first at the joints. However, pressure sores can develop on any area of the body. The standard rule of thumb is to turn a bed patient every two hours, but if you have your loved one at home you will find that turning more frequently is a very small price to pay for being free of pressure sores. Massage any reddened areas when you turn and watch them carefully.

If you are still providing all bedside care there are some tips you should have to avoid problems later on. To avoid pressure sores over the joints on the extremities a quite simple and inexpensive solution is to make "doughnuts" from sanitary napkins and stretch gauze and apply these pads to the elbows, knees, and ankles where they come in contact with the bed or with each other. To be sure, special devices are readily available in medical supply stores but they can be quite costly. To make these pads at home simply form a circle with a sanitary napkin and tape together. Cover this pad with stretch gauze and apply to the joint with more stretch gauze, tightly wrapped enough to be secure but not tight enough to interfere with circulation. Avoid the use of tape on your loved one's skin if at all possible. The skin of the elderly is so fragile that tape can cause breakdown very rapidly. In addition, avoid use of steroid ointment unless prescribed by the physician. This ointment can cause thinning of the skin also.

Learning to turn your loved one in bed, to give a bed bath, and to change the linen with the patient in bed are skills you should learn in a home nursing course. There is a right way and a wrong way to perform each of these actions, and using the wrong method will cause injury to you. Remember to take care of yourself!

If your loved one requires some degree of skilled nursing care and you still wish to keep him or her at home you may employ a temporary nurse to come in for certain periods to do the functions that you are not qualified to do. Quite probably it will be fairly easy for you to learn to do these functions from the nurse if you so desire. Make sure that you employ a reputable agency for these nurses. You may ask your loved one's physician for recommendations or you may be able to check with others in the community who have used an agency's services. Your local hospital may have a home nursing branch as well. Do not hesitate to check the references of the nurses and agency you employ. It is part of your duty as a loving family member to guard your patient from harm.

Again, to return to taking care of yourself, if some aspect of physical caregiving is your "pet peeve" as cutting my mother's toenails is mine, have a professional do it for you. It's worth the extra cost to relieve yourself of this stressor, and you are then free to give your loved one more important emotional support.

Another problem we, as caregivers, sometimes forget is that our loved ones suffer from other diseases as well as one of the dementias. We become so blinded by the disruption to our lives from the dementing illness that we forget such things as diabetes, hypertension, IBD, arthritis, etc. It was brought to my attention that my mother's arthritis was much worse when I brought her home from the nursing home. No, it wasn't the care she received there; it was simply progression of the disease and aging. Without thinking, I had been purchasing blouses that required her to elevate her arms more than was comfortable in order to don them. I had been purchasing slacks that necessitated manual dexterity in fastening the series of zipper and buttons. Her fingers were so twisted that she couldn't manage the finer movements required for buttons.

In making sure she had a balanced diet, I had overlooked the fact that she suffered from hypertension and did not watch for the specially marked "no salt added" cans and boxes in the supermarkets.

Her lower denture had been lost in the nursing home so we had a whole new set of dentures made. I thought she would be able to eat anything she had ever eaten when she had her new dentures. The new dentures did not solve her difficulty in swallowing. Her food must still be either chopped into very small pieces, minced, or pureed. She is overwhelmed by what she perceives as "large" portions. One of my daughters-in-law helped solve that problem by giving me some wonderful child's divided Tupperware plates. The sections are small enough that Mother feels that she can deal with them. They can be refilled as often as needed until she has had an adequate food intake.

We must not become so totally engrossed in caring for the dementia that we ignore the whole person as to tastes, preferences, or fears.

After this discussion it may seem odd to return to more minor matters but the symptoms addressed in the beginning pages of this chapter are those that will require prior preparation on your part during a stage of the disease when you still have time to learn. The following are general tips for health, safety, and peace of mind:

- Pray without ceasing! Ask God to give you the strength and the wisdom to carry out this task.
- Babyproof your home.

- Remove all knives, scissors, and cutting implements from sight. Lock them away if you must. Lock away all poisons, corrosives, etc.
- Remove objects that may become a fall hazard, such as scatter rugs, coffee tables, footstools, etc.
- Remove control knobs from the range and replace them only as needed for preparing meals.
- Make sure no electrical cords are in evidence.
- Get rid of poisonous house plants.
- If your loved one still smokes, make sure you or another responsible party is with him or her at all times when fire-starting implements are in his or her possession. If your loved one is smoking and is a patient with one of the dementing illnesses, he or she will probably not shorten the lifespan too much by being allowed to continue. Having lost so much already, why put your loved one through another stressful and frustrating experience?
- Introduce a walker before it is too late for your loved one to learn to use it. If your loved one is a "wanderer" put keyed dead bolts on the doors so that you can sleep at night.

Other life-normalizing tips:

- A key ring with keys that don't work on anything may soothe a patient who is accustomed to carrying keys.
- Eating a meal in the time normally allotted may overwhelm your loved one. Leave the meal on the table. He or she will return several times to eat portions. Large dinner plates may seem overwhelming when the appetite is poor. Use small dishes and refill as needed.
- If your loved one objects and becomes extremely agitated by being bathed in the shower or tub, remember that he or she is of an age that probably grew up with sponge baths.

You will be able to maintain cleanliness by doing the same. (You may also avoid being injured yourself.)

You may not be able to guard against all hazards, but then neither will a nursing care facility. The laws addressing the use of restraints for the demented specifically advise that they have the same rights to take normal risks as we do.

Remember to take care of yourself. Do not allow yourself to become isolated. Make contacts with other families in your situation. Join a support group if one is available. If not, then think about starting one. If your friends are not emotionally available to you because of their discomfort with dementia, make new friends. If you are in a situation which permits, volunteer to provide respite care for someone else's loved one. Trade "baby-sitting" duties with others who have the same situation. Take care of your health!

Again, take some time for yourself each day. Even if it is only fifteen minutes doing something you enjoy, it will give you strength to go on. I sit on a tree stump in my yard, smoke, and watch the squirrels. The smoking I don't advise—watching squirrels I do. They are so naughty and funny with their antics that you can hardly return to your duties without a smile on your face.

Chapter 17

Moral Judgments:
When Black and White Turn Gray

Moral judgment is an area of care that will give most loving family members of a demented patient more trouble and heartache than any other. I spent months deciding whether this particular chapter belonged in the front of the book or in the back. My final decision was made based on my expectation that you, the reader, will not have reached the end stages of care when you begin to study. I do not pretend to have answers to the questions that will be raised in this chapter. I can only tell you how I handled each issue and why I chose that method. I can only say to you that each of you must make your own choices based on your particular family dynamic and your prayerful study of the subject.

By the time in our lives when we are faced with Alzheimer's disease or any of the other senile dementias, most of us feel that we pretty well have our moral code cast in stone. We are fairly sure that, even if we don't know all the answers, right and wrong will be very easy to distinguish.

I was born and raised in west Tennessee, in the general area where Buford Pusser, the hero of the movie *Walking Tall,* was sheriff. I recall his being asked the question on a television talk show about why he continued his battle against organized crime even after he had been nearly killed and his wife had been murdered.

He looked the interviewer directly in the eye and said, "Well, right's right and wrong's wrong."

In the context in which Buford was speaking this was very true. However, you will soon find as you move through a dementing illness with a loved one that right and wrong are not quite as clear-cut as that.

The first moral issue you will probably face is how much truth you should tell your loved one. My particular family dynamic required the whole truth, I thought. I had never before told my mother an untruth. In the beginning I had no difficulty pursuing this same course. When she inquired about why she was so "muddled" and couldn't remember things, I could quite openly tell her that she was suffering from a dementing illness—perhaps Alzheimer's— and that her memory loss was not her fault but the fault of the disease. I complimented myself on the way I had handled the whole situation without having to tell her an untruth. When she became critically ill and was in the hospital and I realized that she would have to be placed in a skilled nursing facility I simply "wimped out." After my promise to her, made some twenty years in the past, that I would never place her in a nursing home, I could not make my lips form the words to tell her. In addition to my own feelings were my fears that she would be so distressed that she would have a stroke if I told her this particular truth. She had seemed to be able to have light strokes "at will" when she was upset by other things.

I spent the next year and some months carefully referring to the nursing home as "the place where you live now." I never let the words "nursing home" cross my lips in her presence until I had brought her home to stay. Even now, when I need to place her for a few days for respite care, I carefully avoid those words and speak of a nice vacation away from me where she will have nurses to care for her. Am I doing wrong to withhold truth from her which would upset her? I don't know. I only know that I am afraid to take a chance on upsetting her to that degree.

One day Mother asked me, "How's your Daddy?"

She had told everyone for months that she had never been married and had no children. In my surprise at her question I blurted out the truth, that he had been dead since 1974. She did not react that day but on my next visit she became very upset about my having told her that Daddy was dead. Gradually the memory faded and when she asked about him again I simply told her "he's fine." He really is, because he is at home with the Lord, but that wasn't the intent of her question. Did I do wrong to tell her the truth and upset her to that degree? I think so. When she inquires now about why she can't remember things or is doing bizarre things I answer truthfully but in language I know she won't understand. The underlying message is that she is ill and can't help it. She understands that.

Another moral judgment you may be forced to make is just what kind of measures and how long do you wish to have your loved one's life preserved. What quality of life is your loved one experiencing? Is he or she in a chronic vegetative condition with pressure sores? Should you allow nasogastric feeding? IV fluids? What wishes did you ever hear him or her express for this time? If he or she has not expressed any wishes of any kind you are left in a quandary. Even if all the necessary living wills and health care powers of attorney have been completed, you or your loved one may still have a sibling who objects to allowing a natural death. The physician will not generally discontinue heroic measures if there is a family member who resists strongly.

It may come down to your standing alone as the primary caregiver in making life-or-death decisions. Are you strong enough emotionally for this? If not, you must get the family together and try to reach a decision that will be merciful to your loved one, although not necessarily acceptable to all. If no compromise can be reached, the family member with legal control must make the decisions with the help of the health care professionals (have it in writing!). I was very fortunate in that, although my mother refused to put anything on paper, she had expressed her views quite strongly over the years. Most of her views were negative from the perspective of using advanced technology to prolong her life. She always left after visiting a friend or relative in the hospital saying, "Don't you ever let them do that to me."

"That" involved, at various times, nasogastric feeding tubes, stomach pumps, indwelling catheters, and respirators. Her main objection was to being placed in a hospital at all. In her eyes that was almost as bad as being placed in a nursing home.

As most of you know by now, a definitive diagnosis of Alzheimer's disease is practically impossible without an autopsy performed shortly after death. You will probably be asked to give permission to perform such an autopsy when your loved one dies.

If my parents had not expressed firm rejection of the idea of autopsies, I would readily grant permission for one to be performed on my mother, simply so I can say to her descendants, "Yes, she had Alzheimer's." (Or, "No, she didn't have it. It was all those little strokes.")

Unless your loved one has been totally opposed to this procedure, it is recommended. If there is some compelling reason that the family needs to know, you may have to make a judgment contrary to the wishes expressed by your loved one. This is a decision only you can make.

You may feel that in your capacity as primary caregiver you must make sure that your loved one receives everything or has everything withheld that he or she needs to keep him healthy. This may involve withholding a piece of pie from a diabetic, a bag of potato chips from someone with hypertension, cigarettes or a pipe from a smoker, or any of a myriad things that could be harmful to another disease.

Again, this can only be your decision. In caring for my mother, who has hypertension, I do not use any salt at all in cooking, I buy foods with no salt added but I do give her potato chips and cheese puffs. I made this decision because these are her favorite treats and at eighty-six years old and nearing complete helplessness due to dementia, I chose not to deprive her of all that she enjoyed.

She was on a sodium-restricted diet in the nursing home and I stood by and watched her steal a package of crackers from another patient's tray without taking them away from her. I simply told the nurse, after the crackers had been consumed, what had happened so the other patient could have his crackers replaced. I guess this might quite definitely be called a gray area. Not only did I allow her to have something not on her diet orders but had condoned theft. Am I sorry? No. I can't feel convicted for allowing some joy into the life of a person who has lost her personhood.

Long years ago when my father was ill, he developed an aversion to eating. Since he was so thin when he became ill that it was dangerous we tried everything available to medical science to stimulate his appetite. Since he still accepted liquids and the invention of nutritional drinks was still in the future, I made a trip to the next county to buy whiskey (our county was dry) and made him a milkshake daily with a tablespoon of whiskey. Soon the alcohol stimulated his appetite and he was eating again.

My father had been a complete teetotaler, ("lips that touch liquor shall never touch mine") and rigid fundamentalist; this would have been rejected had he known. I never told him, nor did my mother. I've been accused of sinning by causing him to drink an alcoholic beverage when he did not believe in drinking. I felt at the time, and still do, that Paul's admonition to "take a little wine for the stomach's sake" was justification enough for me to keep my father from dying of starvation.

There are very clear areas of morality which we must follow. These are found in the Ten Commandments. I have found none of these to be in conflict with any care I have given to either of my grandmothers, my father, or my mother. Some of the tough decisions we make that give us pause to consider morality are due to cultural patterns and our own family dynamic. If you have been taught that you must always obey your parents you may have problems with the role reversal when you become the parent. If you have always told the absolute, whole truth you will find it difficult to say, "You're really looking good today," when he or she obviously isn't.

We can approach the issue of how much truth if we remember how we dealt with these issues with our own children. When my oldest son was a toddler he asked why Mrs. _____ was getting fat. I told him that she was expecting a baby. He asked if the baby was in her fat tummy. I assured him that it was. He asked no more questions at that time and I gave no more answers. I did not give him a high-school level sex education course. I gave him the information he asked for at the time.

We have to remember that our demented loved ones have lost much of their ability to understand. Too much truth can be extremely confusing. Instead of forcing the truth on a loved one who is having hallucinations, we can enter their fantasy world and work to bring them out. It is far less disturbing to them and easier for us.

At the time my mother was a patient in a nursing home, I became acquainted with a gentlemen there who had been a truck driver prior to retirement and illness. He invited me to go for a ride in his truck. As we sat side by side on the bench he would warn me of upcoming sharp curves and steep hills. I adjusted my posture accordingly. Apparently, in his mind, we were going down a mountain road.

At the end he said, "Well, I've made it down that mountain one more time." I told him what a good driver he was and thanked him for inviting me on his trip. Should I have become combative and insisted that there were no trucks in the unit? Should I have called the nurse and asked for a sedative for him? I think not. It hurt no one for him to relive this memory and to share it with me. I came away knowing more about his early life than I had before and admired him for his abilities. He was happy, I was happy, and a confrontation had been avoided. Think twice before judging everything in black and white.

Chapter 18

Journey's End

I go to prepare a place for you. And if I go and prepare a place for you, I will come again, and receive you unto myself; that where I am, there ye may be also.

John 14:2-3 (KJV)

When first receiving the diagnosis and beginning to absorb its meaning, most caregivers do not immediately realize that their first tentative steps into the valley are probably the beginning of a long, long walk. After all the years my mother and I have been traveling through the valley I fail to remember just when we first received the diagnosis. The walk has been long, arduous, sometimes despairing, and yet there is no end in sight. My mother's overall health seems little changed from that prior to her dementia except for increased arthritis. We may be facing a few days; we may be facing twenty more years.

The realization that this walk may be the longest of our lives can become very depressing if we dwell on it. This is one reason that we face each day and each new problem one day at a time. We do not look ahead for the possibilities of further deterioration. My study of the senile dementias has forewarned me so that I will not be shocked, but I do not spend my days watching for them.

In my morning devotions today, prior to arising to begin a new day with its attendant worries and problems, I was led to study

Isaiah 53:4-5 (KJV) in depth: "Surely he hath borne our griefs, and carried our sorrows: yet we did esteem him stricken, smitten of God and afflicted. But he was wounded for our transgressions, he was bruised for our iniquities: the chastisement of our peace was upon him; and with his stripes we are healed." I realized that in all my years of reading these verses I had only visualized Jesus undergoing all the torture preceding his death on the cross as a sacrifice for our sins. I had not really noticed that He was "afflicted." We are informed elsewhere in the Bible that He suffered every pain that we, His people, suffered. He was afflicted with every disease with which we are afflicted. Did Jesus also take on the burden of Alzheimer's disease? I think He must have. I am led to wonder if Alzheimer's disease was one of the burdens which made His cross so heavy that He fell beneath the load. If this is true, then He understands even more than I had realized just what we are suffering, and His walk through the valley with us is much more significant. The load He helps us bear is a familiar one to Him. Can we as His children envision Him, the Lord of Lords, staggering through the stations of the cross under the load of AIDS, cancer, Alzheimer's disease, Parkinson's disease, etc.?

I continue my study after prayer and find in Isaiah 54:11-12 (KJV) that we who suffer under these afflictions are promised, "O thou afflicted, tossed with tempest, and not comforted, behold, I will lay thy stones with fair colors, and lay thy foundations with sapphires. And I will make thy windows of agates, and thy gates of carbuncles, and all thy borders of pleasant stones." This, then, is the promise of our Lord for our life here on earth and even for our walk through the valley of the shadow of death. We can walk this valley all the way to journey's end with the safe and sure knowledge that God understands and that no matter what the burden we bear from day to day our way is bordered with "pleasant stones."

Journey's End will come, in God's timing. It may come first for my mother. It may come first for me. This I know—that the verse at the beginning of this chapter is true, that we have a place that Jesus has gone to prepare and that He will come Himself to receive us and to usher us into that place designed and built by the Master Builder. We know that our title to that dwelling, beyond this valley, is clear and we look forward with joyous expectation rather than dread for we know that we have been personally escorted through all this by none other than the King of Kings.

We know that we have taken "The Manufacturer's Handbook" as our guide and road map through the valley, and because we have done so, at Journey's End God's promise found in Isaiah 56:12 (KJV) will be our final song:

> For ye shall go out with joy, and be led forth with peace: the mountains and the hills shall break forth before you into singing, and all the trees of the field shall clap their hands.

I have a picture on the wall of my living room which is very precious to me. I was standing in the checkout line of a local discount store when I was struck by this picture on a rack near the front and knew that I must have it. It is a picture of Jesus greeting a saint who is "going home." The head of the homegoing one is on Jesus' shoulder and Jesus is embracing him. The expression on the face of Jesus tells it all: "I am so glad you're home." As there are days when Mother is very unwell physically and I fear that her end may be near, I look at this picture and am able to smile for I realize that when she steps out of this aged and diseased body her mind will once more be clear and sharp and she will recognize the King of Kings as He embraces her in welcome.

Epilogue

My mother's mother had a favorite expression that she used each time I said "I wish"—"If wishes were horses, all beggars would ride." That is so appropriate for my "wish list" for Alzheimer's patients and their caregivers everywhere. "I *wish* . . ."

1. That the cause of this dread disease be discovered *today!*
2. That the cure for this dread disease be discovered *tomorrow!*
3. That no person, anywhere, anytime ever be afflicted with this disease again!

But until then I wish that:

1. All Alzheimer's patients be treated with the dignity due them as God's creations, formed in His likeness.
2. All caregivers be motivated by love—love of God, love for humankind, and love for their patients.
3. The public realize that Alzheimer's is a disease just as cancer, influenza, or any other disease. It is not a failure in moral fiber or a character flaw.
4. It would be understood that there is no one "right" way to deal with Alzheimer's. Each family must determine its own abilities and coping mechanisms.
5. Governmental bodies recognize family care in the home is as valid and cost effective as placement in an institution and reimburse accordingly.
6. Each step in dealing with the disease be as free of bureaucratic rules and regulations as possible.

7. Each caregiver, whether family or institutional, be afforded the help available through support groups.
8. Neighbors and friends of the caregivers be involved in the support groups also so that they may help intelligently.
9. Caregivers, already experienced, volunteer their time and presence to assist new caregivers as they wade through the morass of detail that begins each walk through the valley.
10. Each patient, caregiver, social worker, physician, etc., realize and acknowledge that God is our source of supply, not only of material goods but of comfort, respite, peace, and victory.

I also wish that this volume could have been written in an easier form, in which the reader could pick and choose the exact parts needed at his or her present stage without attempting to absorb all the emotions and pointers at once. Unfortunately, the dementing illnesses do not present themselves as simply as that. Neither do our own responses and emotions. I recall listening to an educator speak on some of the behaviors common to dementias and thinking that life would be so easy if it were all as simple as he made it seem.

Just as the disease suffered by our loved one will present in many forms at many times, our emotions will run the gamut from despair to victory on various days. We find our faith tested over and over. We find that the part of our life we turned over to God yesterday seems to have dropped into our laps again today and we are again attempting to handle it alone. We find the faith we have bragged about when times were good faltering when disaster strikes. We find that living the life of a caregiver, a loving family member, or a caring partner is a test of everything we have ever believed. We find that losing a loved one to a sudden illness and depending on God's grace to bear us up in our grief is so very different from leaning on Him for the long, long miles of this valley. We find that the only instruction we receive from God, "Lean on Me," is the most difficult to follow.

In 1990, when I first admitted that I was suffering from depression, I went to my pastor for counsel. I felt sure that he would give me a list of "Point A, Point B, Point C" to follow, slap me on the forehead and shout "Be healed," and I would go forth leaping with joy. Instead, after listening to me and praying with me, he gave me the wisest counsel I ever received. His answer was "Beth, I believe you need to get some help." It was not long after this conversation and my following his advice that my mother's physician said, "Beth, I'm not saying it's Alzheimer's but . . . you should contact the Alzheimer's support group." Two of the wisest men I have been blessed by knowing have given the same advice—get help.

I believe that God sends the people into our lives who can reach us when we are refusing to listen to Him directly. I still depend on the counsel of these men for help. I depend on the support of my psychiatrist to keep me grounded. I have learned to depend on God for living the everyday-ness of my life with me, which is a much more valuable help than a miracle would be.

Without the help of God (and His servants) I could not have survived the walk through this valley thus far. He has been a constant presence, always there for the thirty-six hours in every day (no that's not a misprint). The family member caring for a loved one with a dementing illness lives at least thirty-six hours in every day and sometimes forty-eight.

Every sign of God's presence has not been of the deeply theological type. I see His hand in the antics of my cat when I awaken feeling very depressed and she comes to play and convince me to get out of bed. Every morning she always does a back-flip out of my bed that is worthy of an Olympic gold medal, turns to me and says *very* forcefully, *Meow!* which means breakfast *now*. I see God in the way two squirrels quarrel over a piece of bread I have put out for them while a blue jay slips in and steals it from both of them.

I especially see His hand in my grandson's being a constant joy in my life, and that just as he graduates and goes out into the world I find that I have another grandchild on the way. Just as one life, so well loved, is descending toward the end, a new life is beginning—another gift from God. I watch my daughter-in-love's face and rejoice in the "pregnancy glow." I watch the little "pooch" on her abdomen and rejoice in its increase in size. I write letters to my unborn grandchild welcoming him or her(?) to this world. Telling him or her(?) how very much love I have waiting. I thank God that He has granted me this gift.

I begin to open my Christmas gifts from my children and buried in the pile I find a gift to "Grandma, from Jack." Jack is my granddog in Florida, a gorgeous chocolate Lab who will play "fetch" with me until we're both ready to drop. I send Jack bags of used tennis balls. My daughter-in-love tells me that he buries his head in the box and is confused by so many balls at once, and I laugh.

I call my daughter-in-love in Memphis and we settle all the world's problems via the telephone.

I see God's hand in the friends who call me on the telephone. One friend and I do book reviews, editorial comments, news analysis, etc., and I feel stimulated, as though I am still a part of the world around me. Another friend and I share laughs all the way from the toes up about some of the antics of the cats, birds, bugs, etc. She owns the house I live in. It was the home of her aunt who had Alzheimer's too. I feel comfortable and at home here. I feel that this house carries a sense of peace and is a safe harbor for AD patients. Her aunt was in the habit of calling us at work to ask what time it was. Now I glance at the clock on the kitchen wall and say, "It's 10:00, Aunt Rosa." No, I don't believe in ghosts, but through my memories Aunt Rosa is still with me. This friend has instituted what she calls "the prayer posse." I call frequently for help from her. She is a mighty prayer warrior as are my other friends.

I know that God placed these friends here long ago, knowing just how much I would need them. I pray that I may, someday, in some way, help them just as they have walked with me through the valley.

We, as Christians, know that Jesus has said, "I will never leave you or forsake you." We know that we can rely on this. We know that no matter how much we love our demented family members and want the best for them that God loves them more. We sense His presence yearning over us as a mother does over her baby. If we listen, we hear Him say, "Come to Me and rest." We, the families of AD patients, become so overwhelmed by the every-day confusion and disruption of our lives that we so easily forget how God loves us and longs to help us. I have to remind myself daily that if He loved me enough to die for me, He surely loves me enough to live with me daily and carry the heavy part of the load.

This, then is my story. Our walk through the valley is not over. I know that harder times may come. I know that my mother may become totally bedridden, incontinent, unable to talk, unable to function at all on her own. I know that this continued walk may be years long. But with that knowledge I have the even surer knowledge that Jesus is with us each step of the way. I know that He will never leave us or forsake us. I know that He has en-camped His angels around us to guard us in all our ways. I know that He will take care, not only of the "small stuff" but of the major problems as they arrive.

On the wall of my bedroom, directly across from my bed, is a picture that I look toward each morning before rising. This pic-ture is of an eagle in flight and Isaiah 40:31 (KJV) is printed above the eagle: "But they that wait upon the Lord shall renew their strength; they shall mount up with wings as eagles; they shall run, and not be weary; and they shall walk, and not faint."

My daily prayer is that I will be able to live this verse, my favorite. That I can run and not be weary, walk and not faint. I know beyond any shadow of doubt that He has renewed my strength over and over again and will continue to do so until we reach the end of the valley when I can see my mother "mount up on wings as eagles" and take her flight to a land where she will be whole, sane, and beautiful once more.

Closing Thoughts

The writings following represent my feelings at different stages during this walk. Some of them are questions, others cries for help. You will find yourself with more of these feelings than can possibly be related in the course of this book.

There will be weeks or months when everything seems to go wrong, followed by more weeks or months when everything is at a standstill. At these times, learning to lean on Jesus is most important for your own sanity.

Research on Alzheimer's disease seems to be progressing at a record pace compared to other diseases such as cancer, AIDS, etc. However, with the graying of America we can expect to see a much greater proportion of our senior citizens developing dementias. It is our part in this war against loss to aid both the ill and those who care for them. A hand up when one is down, a kind word spoken at the checkout, a smile when it is unexpected, can bring help out of proportion to the effort it takes. In the midst of the everyday-ness and acute episodes of rapid degeneration we may be surprised by joy when someone says "Have a nice day"—and means it.

May God speed the day when our medical technology can equate length of life with quality of life.

I Heard My Mother's Voice Again

When I was a child, I suffered from the ordinary "growing pains" of adolescence. I had a king-sized inferiority complex and was always searching for love and approval. I felt somewhere deep inside that my mother loved me but I wasn't mature enough to realize that not everyone can verbalize feelings.

My father's love for me appeared to be completely conditional upon my behavior, so I depended solely on my mother for the security I so badly needed. When going through a particularly bad patch, one of the questions I always asked my mother was "Do you love me?" Her answer was always the same, "Don't be silly; I'm your mother." Not knowing that her care for me as expressed in practical matters was love, I continued to hound her for either a "yes" or a "no." I never received either.

When I had hounded her until she was very frustrated she would tell me, "Stop being silly and go out and play."

"Silly" was my mother's descriptive term for any action or emotion she didn't want to deal with.

Building this phrase into my mental rule book, which consisted of things I would never, never, never say to my children, I proceeded to move on with my life. During the years when I was raising my children I was so busy keeping up with all my never, never, never's that I failed to notice that my mother was losing the voice, the tones with which she scolded me when she said, "Don't be silly."

Our roles in life have been reversed now. Her life is sifting away as sands through an hourglass as she loses more and more of herself to dementia. I am now her parent. I experience many of the same frustrations in dealing with her that she must have had in dealing with me.

During one of our arguments in the early years of her dementia I began with coaxing, then nagging, finally scolding her because she refused to eat.

She said to me, "You don't love me."

Instantly I replied, in tones from the far distant reaches of my memories, "Don't be silly; I'm your daughter." I was brought up short as echoing through the years I heard again, "Don't be silly; I'm your mother."

I heard my mother's voice again that night—and this time she was me.

I Wonder About Alzheimer's

Alzheimer's disease is a progressive, irreversible neurological disorder. Symptoms may include a gradual loss of memory, a decline in the ability to perform routine tasks, impairment of judgment, disorientation, personality changes, difficulty in learning, and loss of language skills. The rate of change varies from person to person.

from Alzheimer's Association—1977

Until my mother's diagnosis several years ago of senile dementia, Alzheimer's type, I was as uneducated about this horrible degenerative disease as most Americans who have not been faced with dealing with a family member with the illness. For the first two years I spent many hours, not only giving her the care she needed as her condition deteriorated, but in learning everything available about the disease, both scientific data and pseudo-scientific musings. It was not until I became physically disabled myself and able to bring her home from the nursing home where she had been placed that we were forced into a one-on-one situation and I began to fully realize the whole truth of my earlier outcries about being given a job description as well as a diagnosis. I learned that even I, her daughter, was attempting to deal with the disease rather than the person. It was then that I began to wonder if there was any connection with the emotional and psychological forces dictated by her former life and the mental fog in which she seemed to exist now.

My mother had always been a loner. Even as a schoolteacher she functioned perfectly intellectually but maintained no emotional ties with either her students or her fellow teachers. In the early years of my childhood before she went outside the home to work, I remembered that most visitors to our home were friends of my father rather than my mother. If she ever had an intimate friend with whom she could share secrets, hurts, joys, I was never aware of it. She and I became emotionally close only after the death of my father. She was not a cold, unloving parent but she seemed, in my childish mind, to go away to a hidden place where she couldn't be reached the minute any unpleasantness arose in our home. She was always in the same room but strangely absent. These periods of absence frightened me, the child, so much that at an early age I took on the task of trying to stand between her and anything that might upset her. I think I had the fear that one day she would "go away" and forget how to come back.

My father was not an abusive man. He was very rigid in his beliefs and held both my mother and myself to extreme codes of dress, manner, and conduct that were dictated by his mother. Since my grandmother lived with us, there was no room for family bonding or personality development except under her eagle eye of disapproval.

My mother had come from a home where constant arguing and bickering were so devastating to her that she had promised herself that when she had a home of her own she would have "peace at any price." She succeeded so well that I only recall one argument between her and my father during my entire life with them. After that argument she was "away," not speaking to anyone, for several days and my father convinced me that it was all my fault. I determined then that I would never allow that to happen again. I was seven years old at the time.

During the intervening years while she went back to college, obtained her degree and teaching credentials, and taught fourth grade, I was married and away from everyday observation of her behavior. I still noticed on visits home that she seemed very distant. I interpreted this as anger against me for having left her to cope alone. I never realized the depth of withdrawal from painful emotions she was practicing. She had maintained her assigned role as "messenger" of my father's orders in his attempts to insinuate that she "ruled the roost." The relationship I had developed with my father allowed me to see through the ruse so I felt even more responsible for helping her stay "fixed" in the here and now.

She took an early retirement to care for my father when his dementia required twenty-four-hour supervision. He had sustained severe brain damage in an automobile accident.

Now, through hindsight, I can see that his dementia began long before the accident. After three years of exhausting, laborious care for him with only myself and my husband and children to assist her, he died. At this time she was free to be herself but the habits of so many years were not so easily broken. When we began to share a home, I not only carried on long conversations with her about the present, but encouraged her to remember her life and to express her feelings about things that had happened to her in her earlier years. It was during these years that she told me repeatedly that when faced with something emotionally painful she "just put it out of her mind." I understood that this was what I had seen as "going away." I, the eternal rebel, asked many times "why didn't you say, do, act?" only to be told again that she just put it out of her mind and forgot about it.

When she began to exhibit signs of approaching dementia, I tried even harder to keep her interested in her life as it was now. Looking back, I can see signs even earlier than I thought at the time that she was indeed "going away." She became compulsive about locked doors and windows. Every door and window had to be checked and rechecked before going out, returning home, or going to bed. We had a constant running battle because she nailed the windows shut as I followed close behind removing the nails.

At last she has indeed "gone away" and forgotten how to return. More and more information is being lost from her memory banks every hour of every day. While the medical community is desperately searching for a cause and a cure, we family members are holding on desperately to each little bit we see of her personality. The only skills she maintains constantly are her socialization skills. She still greets everyone she meets with a big smile and a "Good morning; how are you today?"—the typical skills learned in the cradle of Southern womanhood.

Now that she has regressed in stages through her early years and is a child again, needing directions for the simplest tasks, I am left to wonder if the deterioration of her brain cells is wholly a function of organic disease or if her years of denial of all painful emotion created a fertile ground for the disease process to advance more quickly.

I am also left to wonder if the fact that I carry her genes and have also responded inappropriately to painful episodes in my own life will bring me to this same loss of personhood earlier than I anticipated. Will the psychotherapy I am undergoing perhaps give me a few more years or even months of sanity? Or is it too late even now?

I wonder about Alzheimer's.

Waiting

Mother "feels bad" today. She has difficulty explaining just what her symptoms are. I check her blood pressure—it's fine. I listen to her heart and hear a strong beat but a definite arrhythmia. I check her radial pulse, again strong but faltering. She is more confused. She finally shows me that she hurts at her collarbone. Is this another TIA, sore throat, or is she having a heart attack? I dare not check her carotid pulse. I know I will feel disruption of the blood flow. I'm waiting, watching.

I ask her if she would like a drink. She says no. I tell her she should lie down. She agrees. This is not normal. She doesn't lie down in the daytime. The cats realize something is not normal. Widget sits on the foot of Mother's bed watching her intently. Tat sits on the cedar chest watching also. I cannot sit. I wander from room to room and back again. I'm waiting, watching.

My mind and my heart are in conflict. My mind tells me that this is the way she would prefer it. My mind reaffirms all the instructions she has given me over the years. My memories tell me that she wanted to die at home, in her own bed. My heart cries out, "no, no!" Call the doctor, call the ambulance! Mother, hold on! One more day, one more hour.

I want to place one of my nitroglycerin tablets under her tongue. She won't allow it. I want someone to sit with me as I wait and watch. I know that no one can leave work, leave housework undone, drop everything, to come for what may be a false alarm. I know that I must bear this burden with Christ as my only companion and comforter. I wait and watch.

I realize that I am also in conflict within my mind. Part of me longs for the freedom I've never had. The freedom to be, to grow, to learn. Part of me holds onto the bondage that has defined me and my place in the world. Part of me longs for the freedom to soar, while part holds on desperately to the "nest" of habit. I wait and watch.

Today may not be the day after all. She may rally many times yet but for today the pain has finally broken through all the wise judgments and promises made, and I am grieving. I grieve for the seven years we have traveled this valley. I grieve for the previous years when we couldn't communicate. I realize that in my innermost heart I have longed for a miracle. I have longed to exchange all the years of pain for a few short years when she can be truly mother and I can be truly daughter without the filter of father, grandmother, and others standing between. I have wished for a time when she could say "yes" or "no" to a request of mine without asking permission herself first. I have waited and watched in vain. It's too late.

Realization has struck that the "tomorrow when I will think about it" has come. This is the "tomorrow" I had used as an emotional credit card, against which I had charged all the pain and sense of loss. Tomorrow has become today and still I wait and watch.

Some years ago, I looked into her eyes and realized that I was watching her die, one brain cell at a time. I look into her eyes today and see, not only the used up, burned-out brain cells, but the encroaching physical blindness. She has been tested. There is no help for her eyes. I move very close so that she can see me. She no longer recognizes my voice. I watch and wait.

We stumble together through our days, days spent on the mechanics of physical care, days spent soothing frightening emotions, days spent watching and waiting.

Losing my mother is something that happened when the plaques and tangles began to consume her brain. I watch as all my yesterdays disappear, with hers, under the plaques and tangles. I know I must give up but keep trying desperately to force memories. Memories of my friend who called her "Auntie Mom" and told her he had "taken great joy" in seeing her. He lost his life in an automobile accident at an early age and never had to watch his father disappear as my mother has. Somehow I think he would still sit quietly, then say, "I've taken great joy in seeing you." She doesn't remember. I watch and wait.

"Mother" is gone. This person I care for is a stranger moving about in her body. She is a stranger even to herself. She repeats her name several times daily to reassure herself that she still exists. I watch and wait.

Even though Mother is gone, when I look at the loved and familiar body, I see family resemblances. I see expressions familiar to me. I tell her how she looks like "Aunt Donie" now. She doesn't know who I look like for she can't remember who I am.

I wonder as I wait, "Will I disappear when her body dies?" In some deep part of me there is a core that believes, in spite of all rational thinking, that when she is well and truly gone, her ashes buried beside my father, then I will no longer exist. My life has been spent in service. Will I be able to transfer that service to others? I have waited upon the Lord, He has renewed my strength to finish this course, but still I wonder if I am but a chimera, sent here to care for these children who were my parents. I wait and watch—and I am afraid.

Today

The deterioration continues. Sometimes it moves so fast that I am caught unaware; sometimes it moves on snail's feet. Some days she is incontinent and I wonder if we have reached the last stage. Then after two days of attempts at retraining, she is no longer incontinent. I am confused. I still imagine the giant ameobic entity perched on top of her brain with pseudopods ever lengthening. I become frustrated, for part of me wants so desperately to believe that she could help herself in some way.

There are days when I would prefer to stay in bed with my head covered rather than arise to face all the decisions needed. When I would simply make myself a peanut butter sandwich, I must decide on and prepare a balanced diet for her. I must choose her clothing for the day, for she is too confused to do so. I must assess her condition today as opposed to yesterday's. I must decide when its time to see her physician. Sometimes she tells me she is in pain but can't tell me where. Some mornings she sleeps later than normal and I tiptoe into her room to make sure she is breathing. On other occasions she wakes me at 2:00 a.m. and refuses to go back to bed.

I wonder about asking to be tested myself. I wonder if the tests are definitive enough to be valid yet. I wonder if I could handle hearing that I will become demented also. I decide that I will wait until after her death to be tested.

I am afraid that I would not be able to continue to care for her if I knew that I were beginning the ten- to twenty-year presymptom stages. I give in to that fear and wait.

Friends tell me of remedies they have read about all the way from ginseng to Vitamin E. We did the Vitamin E trials years ago. There are no magic pills. We try the new ginkgo biloba in exceedingly small doses but find that it causes more extreme agitation and sleep disturbances. I decide to stop experimenting, yet I know that I will continue to follow the research and be ready to attempt anything that just might help. I am not ready yet to admit defeat.

Someday the amoeba will find its way to the cells that control the memory of how to breathe or the memory that causes the heart to beat. Will there be grief at that stage? I feel that I have grieved already but wonder about the silence in the home without her latest personality.

This one thing I know, that as we have walked through the valley of the shadow of death we have had a constant companion in Jesus Christ. For this reason I will fear no evil for He will continue to be with me, just as always, exactly at the point of my need.

As we continue the walk with its days of agitation, irritability, and memory loss, I realize even more that the Comforter did come just as Jesus promised before his ascension and that as I face new problems daily Jesus still advises "don't sweat the small stuff," while the Holy Spirit continues, "it's all small stuff." I realize that love and care are the only truly important facets of this walk. I realize too that I have been given a gift in my opportunity to learn from her and about other patients and their families. I realize that we need to share our stories, share our joys and sorrows, and uphold each other until the time when this disease is conquered.

Each of us who has walked this valley has a story to tell. These stories may someday lead to the very idea the researchers need. At the very least, sharing our stories, sharing our faith, and holding one another's hands through the tough spots binds us together in human love. We must share the knowledge that until the researchers are successful, God's grace is sufficient and His grace is greater than all our fears.

God speed the researchers and God speed our understanding.

Fighting Back

When we first begin our study of dementing illness, we see that we are faced with a long, long road, progressively more difficult, until at last our loved one goes home to be with the Lord. Viewing the road ahead is frightening, depressing, and filled with trouble. In looking at these features and realizing just what we face it is easy to fall into an acceptance of the disease, focus on its terminal nature, and look no farther.

There is light at the end of the tunnel. Researchers are focusing daily on finding a cause for these life-robbing diseases. They may find that there is no single root cause for the diseases, but a combination of factors that, taken together, cause the brain to cease its proper function. Many other diseases are a function of the breakdown of the immune system from a multitude of causes. Why not dementia?

Those of us who do "hands on" care of patients with AD or the other dementing illnesses may have knowledge of prior problems in the patient's life that may have contributed to this final stage. Through networking with one another, with patients in early stage AD, and with physicians and researchers, we may be able to add that one little piece of information that will be the stimulus to put it all together and develop a clearer understanding.

We know that finding a cure or a treatment that will delay onset or progression of the disease depends almost entirely on finding the root causes. This is where we laypersons can be of most value.

Because I care for my mother, I am the one who is able to tell her physician that she has always avoided dealing with frightening or unpleasant emotions. I am the one who is able to trace at least four generations of the women in her family who have suffered from early-onset hypertension. I am the one who knows that both her brother and a first cousin suffer from Parkinson's disease. I am the one who knows that her mother suffered from dementia for many years prior to her death from a massive stroke. If there were other details of her history and family health history I would be the one who knew of them. I have information he needs to put together a definitive diagnosis. Each family caregiver has information that is known only within the family. This information should be relayed to the physician as early as possible. We make the mistake in many instances of believing that because our loved one has been treated by many physicians that his or her medical records will be complete without our input. This feeling is probably wrong. One of the greatest problems in treating the aged has been that they were being cared for by a variety of specialists and rarely have they informed each specialist of the medications they are given by other physicians. As the family member most concerned with the care of our demented loved one, we must make sure that we have all the information and pass it on to the primary care physician.

I have given my primary care physician all the information about my medical history and family medical history that I remembered. I cannot be sure that I have remembered each illness or each treatment. Should I become demented it would be my children who would be able to tell my physician that I suffered an acute allergic reaction to ergotamine and that its vasoconstrictive action left me with permanent circulatory damage. It will be my children who can relay the information that I began having seizure disorders and hypertension prior to age forty and that my mother's family had a history of hypertension while my father's family suffered from migraine headaches and seizure disorders. One little piece of this information might point him in just the exact direction to recognize some causal relationship.

While we, as loving family members, need to give up the worries and cares to a loving God to help us with bearing our burdens, we must never give up the fight against the disease. It may be too late to help our loved one, but we could provide needed information to researchers.

We, as loving family members, friends, and support groups must never give up the fight. We are not simply fighting death in this battle. We are fighting the death of the self while the body continues to function. We are fighting the loss, the confusion, the financial devastation, the destruction of family relationships.

With the cost of medical care at an all-time high, with the take-over of managed health care, with the budget cuts for health care, we realize that there will be less funds for drugs, for nursing home beds, for needed hospitalization as America ages. With the graying of America bringing on the increase of patients with senile dementias, the availability of health care has to suffer. The only answer to this problem is either a cure or some treatment for delaying onset and disease progression.

Even as I was writing this portion one of the major nursing home corporations in the United States announced its intention to phase out its Medicaid patients and take only those with the ability for private payment. This will place nursing home care beyond the reach of a large percentage of patients suffering from dementia. This is only the beginning. New methods of care must be devised as well as continued research into the biological causes and treatments. Families will be faced with complete financial destitution and be forced to care for their loved one at home or to sacrifice their own financial security, their children's college funds, etc., to meet the challenge of these disabling diseases.

We are not alone in this fight. I am reminded of an old hymn sung in my church when I was a child. "I heard the voice of Jesus, telling me still to fight on. He promised never to leave me, never to leave me alone."

Giving our worries and cares to Him, depending on His grace to support us, we can also depend on His presence and His guidance in fighting back against this devastating illness. He promised never to leave us alone.

We must stay on the battlefield. Retreat is not an option. We, the loving family members are the foot soldiers, in the trenches. With God's help, with the dedication of the medical establishment and the researchers, we will win this battle.

We Must!

Final Prayer

Our loving heavenly Father, grant your peace to our loved ones suffering from these most dreadful diseases. Shine the light of Your great love through the fog that exists in their minds. Even though they may have lost their memories of You, in Your infinite grace give them rest from their fears.

Give us, their loving caregivers, the patience, the fortitude, and the peace we need for respite from the burdens of our everyday lives. Let Your love shine forth through us to our loved ones and to the thousands of others like them. Let us build bridges of love and hope between families going through the same turmoil. Teach each of us that our blessed Savior, Jesus Christ, is always with us, that He came to bear our burdens and share our sorrows. Help us to give up our worries and cares and to realize at all times that Your everlasting arms are underneath. Help us to remember that Your blessed Holy Spirit will be with us and comfort us through our trials.

We ask this in the Name above all other Names, Jesus Christ, our Lord. Amen.

Recommended Reading

Cheney, Marshall (September 1996). Keeping Depression at the Door. *Los Angeles Alzheimer's Association Newsletter.*

Duke Family Support Program Quarterly Newsletter. The Caregiver.

Gruetzner, Howard (1988). *Alzheimer's: A Caregiver's Guide and Sourcebook.* New York: John Wiley and Sons, Inc.

Holy Bible—Reader's preferred version.

Koenig, Harold, G., Lamar, Tracy, and Lamar, Betty (1997). *A Gospel for the Mature Years.* Binghamton, NY: The Haworth Pastoral Press.

Lynch, David (1994). *He Giveth More Grace.* Nashville, TN: Star Song Publishing Group.

Mace, N. and Rabins, P. (1991). *The 36 Hour Day.* Baltimore, MD: The Johns Hopkins University Press.

National Alzheimer's Association Quarterly Newsletter. Advances.

Rankin, Peg (1994). *How to Care for the Whole World and Still Take Care of Yourself.* Nashville, TN: Broadman and Holman Publishers.

Stafford, Florence (1986). *Caring for the Mentally Impaired Elderly.* New York: Henry Holt and Company.

Index

Order Your Own Copy of
This Important Book for Your Personal Library!

CARING FOR A LOVED ONE WITH ALZHEIMER'S DISEASE
A Christian Perspective

_____ in hardbound at $49.95 (ISBN: 0-7890-0872-6)

_____ in softbound at $18.95 (ISBN: 0-7890-0873-4)

COST OF BOOKS_____	☐ **BILL ME LATER:** ($5 service charge will be added) (Bill-me option is good on US/Canada/Mexico orders only; not good to jobbers, wholesalers, or subscription agencies.)
OUTSIDE USA/CANADA/ MEXICO: ADD 20% _____	
POSTAGE & HANDLING_____ (US: $3.00 for first book & $1.25 for each additional book) Outside US: $4.75 for first book & $1.75 for each additional book)	☐ Check here if billing address is different from shipping address and attach purchase order and billing address information.
	Signature _____
SUBTOTAL_____	☐ **PAYMENT ENCLOSED: $** _____
IN CANADA: ADD 7% GST_____	☐ **PLEASE CHARGE TO MY CREDIT CARD.**
STATE TAX_____ (NY, OH & MN residents, please add appropriate local sales tax)	☐ Visa ☐ MasterCard ☐ AmEx ☐ Discover ☐ Diner's Club
FINAL TOTAL_____ (If paying in Canadian funds, convert using the current exchange rate. UNESCO coupons welcome.)	Account # _____ Exp. Date _____ Signature _____

Prices in US dollars and subject to change without notice.

NAME _____

INSTITUTION _____

ADDRESS _____

CITY _____

STATE/ZIP _____

COUNTRY _____ COUNTY (NY residents only) _____

TEL _____ FAX _____

E-MAIL_____
May we use your e-mail address for confirmations and other types of information? ☐ Yes   ☐ No

Order From Your Local Bookstore or Directly From
The Haworth Press, Inc.
10 Alice Street, Binghamton, New York 13904-1580 • USA
TELEPHONE: 1-800-HAWORTH (1-800-429-6784) / Outside US/Canada: (607) 722-5857
FAX: 1-800-895-0582 / Outside US/Canada: (607) 772-6362
E-mail: getinfo@haworthpressinc.com
PLEASE PHOTOCOPY THIS FORM FOR YOUR PERSONAL USE.

BOF96